Lose Weight

Not Strength

Kick start your weight loss habits naturally

By RICK ALVES

Lose Weight Not Strength

Kick start your weight loss habits naturally

About the Author

I have been using the diet techniques for more than ten years now. As a weight loss expert, it is my goal to help others who are interested in using the diet for the first time or looking for new ways to lose weight, so I'd like to share my knowledge with you.

Losing weight is not an easy task, one of the many reasons why you find yourself struggling with that concept day in and day out. There is no easy way out of this; however, it is not impossible to do either. All you have to do is open your mind to the possibility of working a little harder to incorporate some healthy lifestyle choices in your daily routine. Yes, that's pretty much it.

I have been through what you're going through right now, and as time goes by things do get easier than they are now. The first few months will be hard, but then there will come a time when you're healthy, thin and fit and wouldn't know what else there is to life than being healthy. The secret to being thin is not starving yourself or working out until your muscles collapse; the secret is way simpler. Read on and find out what it is you need to do – to be successful at losing weight.

Join our mailing list and get updates on new releases, free mini-courses, and new recipes we introduce from time to time based on our research. Click here to sign up or visit our website www.puredietweightloss.com/newsletter.

Special Gift for Readers

Throughout the book, there are numerous mentions of additional resources that can help you through this journey. You can get all these valuable resources by visiting our website www.puredietweightloss.com

You can also join our mailing list and get updates on new releases, free mini-courses, and new recipes we introduce from time to time based on our research. Click here to sign.

Introduction

Who doesn't want to be smart and healthy? Nowadays, weight loss is the number one concern for millions of people around the world who remain unhappy with the way they look and feel. Even though it is very easy to gain a few extra pounds, losing the same is one of the hardest tasks you can be confronted with. Hard and soft fat are both nightmares for dieters who often spend large amounts of money only to get back in shape.

Remember the generous portion of turkey you had for thanksgiving? The amazing walnut pie that you couldn't stop eating on New Year's Eve? Yes, it is all these festive eating habits that usually bring individuals to a point where gaining additional weight is no longer an option, and neither is losing weight because the pain attached to it is just unbearable.

What then, is the solution to obesity and those hard wired diet plans that seem to be leading you nowhere? Years of research, both in medical and nutritional spheres, have led to a lot of understanding of how the body works when a dieter starts a weight loss program. Based on this knowledge, many new weight loss tips and strategies have been designed which lead to successful trimming of fat reserves in the body.

This information guide is written for the purpose of helping dieters lose weight and maintain it thereafter. Since, many of you would be highly frustrated right now because of the lack of results from the diet and exercise plan, this book is for you and all those who need a rich resource for guidance in this matter. Remember, weight loss may be hard, but when you set your mind to it, it is by no means impossible.

The foundation of this book lies in a simple rule which is the crux of every well planned diet regime. According to this Golden Rule, the amount of calories you burn every day should be more than the amount you need on a daily basis. Fulfilling this rule automatically means that you are out of the evil clutches of obesity and on your way to a healthier self.

While it does sound easy in theory, making sure that you burn more than you gain requires a change in lifestyle. You cannot be sitting at your desk for the better part of the day (not to forget the Big Mac meal you ordered for lunch!) and then expect to lose weight. This is the equation for weight gain, not loss. Therefore, the sooner you want to lose weight, the sooner you need to start accepting change.

This book is the perfect resource to explore the 'change' and introduce it in your life in a very healthy manner. Weight loss requires a mix of psychological, physical and emotional stimulants- all of which are triggered by various life situations.

Taking control of your life and evaluating the path it is taking is the best way to ensure a healthier mind and body.

The Extra Inches: What Am I Doing Wrong

Something's wrong with My Weight Measuring Machine

At the sight of the numerals on your weighing scale, what is the first thought that comes to mind? If you are one of those who head out to buy a new weighing machine, thinking this one is broken, it is time to get a reality check. While your machine may really be broken (how long has it been since you bought it?), blaming it for making the added layers of fat prominent isn't really fair, is it?

Perhaps the biggest problem with most obese people is that they can't resist the sight of food. For them, food is a way to enjoy life and become happy. As they go on eating, Christmas after Christmas, obese people literally get 'drugged' and before they know it, it's too late. Since the problem with obesity and constant eating is more psychological than physical, overweight individuals have to do way more than simply cut back on their intake.

With the psychological twist in the equation, the entire argument on obesity takes a new turn. For the longest time, it was thought that those who end up getting obese do so because of their own faults. Contrary to this belief, psychologists assert that no matter how hard obese individuals try, they cannot stop binging unless they are guided and counseled.

Are You Eating More Than You Should?

There have been several large scale studies conducted in America that show a very clear picture of the way eating habits and lifestyles have changed over the last ten decades or so. Many of these surveys first conducted in 1890s reported a mean average weight of 145-150 pounds for women and 165-170 pounds for men.

From this time to the mid-1970s, these weight averages were quite representative of both genders, indicating that there were no major changes introduced into their lives. However, from the mid-1970s onwards, a 25% increase in weight for both genders has been recorded by several reputable studies conducted to gauge health standards.

To match this study with calorie intake, a further research was conducted that revealed that in 1965, the average calories consumed by a typical American numbered close to 3100. The same number has now jumped up to 3900, with everything else constant. These results pose a very pressing question: Are we meeting more than we need?

Certainly, if the people in 1965 could survive with 800 less calories, so can we. However, this question begs an answer, since a solution to the fight against obesity can possibly be derived from it. It is obvious that people today eat more unhealthy foods than their counterparts did some 40 years back. But why is this so?

According to many nutritionists, people are eating more today because they have become addicted to processed sugars and fat. This addiction is directly traced to the way our brain controls our desire for food. Let's take some biology into account at this point, because understanding the reasons of why we eat more today than we did yesterday have a lot to do with how our brain coordinates with the rest of the body.

The Biological Aspect Of Weight Gain

The body needs two essential types of oils called Omega 6 and Omega 3. Both these compounds have to be present in a very delicate balance because they are needed in a 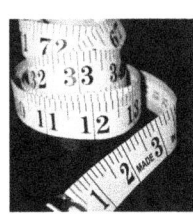 fixed quantity by the body for essential procedures like the building of the outermost layer of red and white blood cells. In their correct quantities, both, Omega 6 and Omega 3 are highly beneficial. However, it is when the balance tips that the brain's control over food dysfunctions.

Omega 6 is derived from oils that are very saturated, while Omega 3 is taken in by consuming less saturated oils. With the inclusion of heavily processed foods in our diets, the level of Omega 6 in the body has increased drastically- to a point that it now affects the brain's power over food desire. Here's how it works: appetite controlling cells in the Hypothalamus- a nerve packed part of the brain- have a rich supply of receptors that are made of a naturally occurring form of Omega 6. Hence, when Omega 6 increases in the body with the consumption of processed foods, there is a proportional increase in the appetite control receptors, which consequently lead an individual to feel hungrier.

The ultimate result? Body becomes susceptible to eating disorders.

What Are Eating Disorders

Eating disorders are complicated dietary conditions that result from a variety of psychological, social and physical factors. People suffering from Eating disorders are known to use food as a 'tool' to cope with unpleasant feelings,

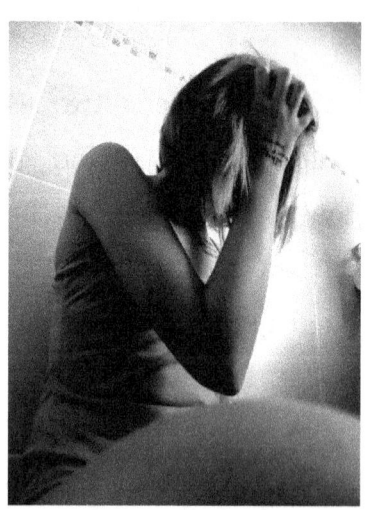

situations and circumstances. Instead of eating to survive, they survive to eat.

Therefore, eating disorders are overwhelming for an obese individual because even if he doesn't want to binge, he is forced to do so by an uncontrollable urge to feel better in depressing and overly stressful situations.

There are many reasons because of which these disorders surface. Some of the most prominent ones are:

- Psychological Factors
  - Extremely low Self Esteem that makes a person feel really bad about how he looks how he feels or how he behaves.
  - Insecurities about life that lead them to believe they do not belong anywhere and that they do not have any control over life.
  - Loneliness, depression, anxiety and stress

- Interpersonal Factors
  - Unstable relationship with parents, partners or friends
  - An overwhelming history of being abused, teased or bullied
  - History or sexual abuse

- Being unable to express emotions and feeling suffocated

- Social Factors

  - Societal definitions of how thin a man or woman should be
  - Peer pressure of having the perfect body and being very cautious of eating habits
  - Cultural norms that place value on individuals based on the way they look
  - Discrimination, prejudice and judgments about overweight and obese people who find it hard to fit in the crowd

- Biological Factors

  - Many types of eating disorders are in family genetics. If parents are obese and have an uncontrolled eating habit, then there is a high probability that the children will follow similar patterns of behavior.

Diseases That Cause Obesity

Apart from eating disorders, another primary reason for obesity is the increasing instance of several serious and fatal diseases. Of the 65 million adults that are morbidly obese, a huge chunk suffers from these diseases which make an individual overweight and prevent him or her from reducing weight, despite a perfectly functional diet and exercise plan in place. Even though gradual monitoring and control of the ailments help patients put a stop to weight gain, there is often no permanent cure that can be looked forward to as a remedy to lifetime obesity.

Since diseases are another cause of being overweight, many a times, eating disorders worsen if an individual has such a disease that he finds difficult to cope up. In this case, the disease and its effects make the individual highly insecure, resulting in a low self-esteem that eventually leads to binging and uncontrolled desires to find solutions to life problems with food.

The following are the top diseases that lead to weight gains.

1. **Arthritis-** Severe arthritis limits the movements of individuals on a daily basis. In many cases, people are instructed by doctors to not even walk around the house because the simplest of activities result in unbearable pain in joints, particularly those of knees and toes. With reduced activity, weight gain becomes inevitable.

2. **Plantar Fasciitis-** Plantar Fasciitis is a painful condition of the underside of the foot and the heel. It is characterized by the structural breakdown of the bone and ligament connection on the sole of the foot that leads to extreme pain when the patient walks. If this discomfort continues, patients end up in sedentary positions for the most of the day, which makes weight gain a high possibility.

3. **Dysthymia-** Dysthymia is acute and chronic depression that is characterized by years of hopelessness and negativity that takes over a person's life. Unlike episodes of depression, Dysthymia doesn't come and go; it is a condition that becomes second nature to the patient. As a result of this condition, those affected by it binge on food to relieve stress.

4. **Hypothyroidism-** Hypothyroidism is a condition that affects the ability of the thyroid gland to produce thyroid hormones. In the absence of these necessary hormones, the body is unable to carry out essential functions, the regulation of energy from food consumption being the biggest problem. As a result of this, a Hypothyroidism patient suffers from an unintentional gain of several pounds that greatly reduce the quality of life.

5. **Menopause-** Menopause marks the end of the menstrual cycle in women. During menopause, bodily hormones change to a great extent, resulting in many symptoms like hot flashes, loss of sleep and dryness of the vagina. Another prominent effect of menopause is weight gain as a result of the changes of the internal environment of the body. Women going through menopause are strictly advised to watch what they eat on a regular basis.

6. **Cushing Syndrome-** The most prominent symptom of the Cushing Syndrome is an upper body weight gain that makes it hard for patients to perform daily chores with ease. This disease is a result of high levels of the hormone Cortisol that leads to severe conditions like painful stretch marks, weakness and glucose intolerance.

7. **Polycystic Ovarian Syndrome-** Polycystic Ovarian Syndrome is characterized by the presence of benign masses on the ovaries. These masses are a result of a high imbalance of sex hormones, namely, estrogen and progesterone in women which cause sudden and unintentional weight gain. This is usually hard to shed because the hormones need to be stabilized for fat to burn.

Is my desk Job the Culprit?

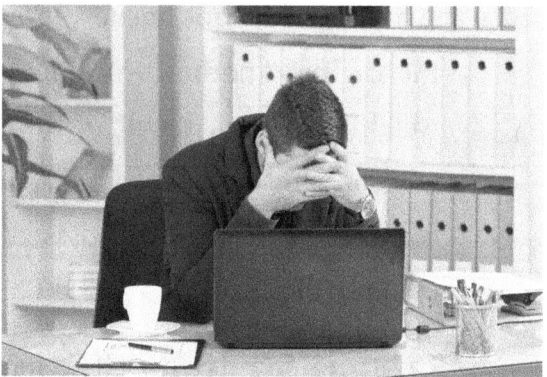

When looking into the reasons why your body is unable to lose weight, there are several arrows that all point in different directions. Digging out one particular cause is often hard because it requires a thorough scanning of your lifestyle choices and the many ways you treat and mistreat your body. However, one particular reason that is often quoted by many nutritionists and gym instructors is the lack of activity in people's lives, which is a direct cause of obesity and the diseases related to it.

If you think you are gaining weight because of the sedentary job you have, you are not alone. According to several studies, people who are very inactive during work hours are 41% more prone to weight gain than their active counterparts. Such research reveals that a 9-5 job is, perhaps, the biggest reason why you may not be losing weight despite following a diet plan staunchly.

Moreover, the same studies also conclude that within the span of only 2 to 3 hours that an employee spends sitting, levels of good cholesterol decrease by 20% in the body and the risk of diabetes increases drastically. Moreover, while doing work in a sedentary position, you tend to burn 50% less calories than you would while moving around.

With so much data to back up this claim, individuals who have sedentary jobs often find themselves in a fix. Jobs related to administrative work, IT development, and legal paperwork, engineering, designing and teaching are some of the most notorious ones that are associated with weight gains. And there's more! When you end up sitting around a desk all day long, the chances of munching on unhealthy snacks are way higher as well!

Is there a solution to this problem that doesn't involve quitting your desk job? Luckily for you there is. However, this solution largely depends on how motivated you feel to bring a change to your lifestyle and to stay healthy. To make sure you break the spell of long sitting hours, experts suggest that you make your own work schedule for moving around.

For instance, instead of taking a cab for the last block home, sprint the distance to pump some energy in your legs. Instead of taking the elevator, how about taking the stairs to the third floor? Instead of calling the guy from the copy room, walk your way to the copy machine itself? It is these small changes that can help you introduce changes to a sedentary lifestyle at no cost- but with a truckload of benefits.

Moreover, since this problem has been recognized by the management of big organizations as well, a trend to promote a healthy lifestyle at work has begun with a lot of enthusiasm. Getting fresh fruit baskets for all employees and departments is one of the most praiseworthy shifts made by organizations which try to show their workers that their health matters to them.

Similarly, apart from having fresh and healthy fruits during work hours, different managements make it a point to educate desk staff on the importance of moving about- even if it is to take a stroll till the gallery and get some fresh air!

What Am I Doing Wrong?

What is it that you are not doing to lose weight? If you have set your mind to lose the extra holiday weight or finally make a move from obesity towards a healthy and wealthy lifestyle, shouldn't you be making daily progress?

Many a times, it becomes hard to shed even a single pound, let alone record drastic changes in your figure within a month or two of your fat shredding plan. Such slow and sluggish results are the best de-motivators and are often enough to demoralize a dieter to an extent that he leaves the regime midway- only to return to binging and causing harm to his body.

According to trainers, the question 'What am I doing wrong?' is one of the most frequent queries they get from trainees who want to lose fat and at the same time maintain a strong and healthy body. While this question does not have an easy answer, if you are one of these people who have had immense trouble following a diet plan because of the lack of results, there's a lot you can do to make sure all your effort are not in vain.

The first step is to understand the difference between weight loss and fat loss. While it is usually used interchangeably, many nutritionists prefer to draw a line between the two because it leads to a clearer idea of how to get in shape. Fat loss is the shedding of extra pounds of fat that collect around organs, making an individual look chubby.

Essentially, everyone aims to lose fat because they want to maintain the strength of the body by building up on muscle fibers. A very raw attempt to sum up this difference would be to say that weight includes fat and muscles; while the fat is only the 'chubbiness' that you want to get rid of.

Once this is understood, the next step is to break-down the Fat Loss Process. How can pounds of fat be lost and kept off permanently? Does it mean you should never eat what you like? Or does it mean you should spend every minute of your free time exercising? Gladly, staying healthy and losing weight is not such a hard process that robs you of pleasure time.

However, without adequate knowledge, no amount of efforts will reap results- which is why understanding what initiates fat loss is a top priority for dieters. This information is thus extremely important to help you get past the hurdles that are hindering you from getting an ideal body.

The Fat Loss Trio

For an effective fat loss program, the Fat Loss Trio should be kept in mind. This Trio presents a combination of the three most important elements 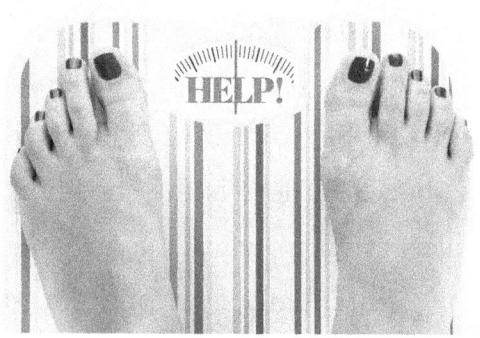 that should be incorporated into just about any weight loss program. If one of these elements is out of place, losing weight can become a hard nut to crack!

The Fat Loss Trio includes:

1. A well thought out diet

2. Healthy habits

3. Effective exercises

Every time you kick-start a new plan, make sure you have these elements in an eloquent balance so that even the smallest effort towards getting fit results in a reward. Even though each of these three elements overlap and are interlinked because the weight loss plan is a combination of all; they have been mentioned separately to clearly lay out the concepts for the reader.

1. The Ultimate Weight Loss Diet Plan

Remember the Golden Rule of fat/weight loss? We discussed in the introductory paragraphs that weight loss is all about the right diet that manages calorie count effectively. For you to bring any change to your body, it is essential that you keep the Golden Rule in mind.

Weight loss = Calories Eaten < Calories Burnt

Everything about a diet plan revolves around burning calories. Calories are energy units that you gain by consuming a variety of foods- all of which have different calorie counts. When a dieter starts a weight loss regime, he has to restrict himself to a certain level of calorie intake per day. Depending on how obese an individual is and the amount of fat that needs to be shed, calorie intake differs from person to person.

For those who seek the help of professional trainers, it is much easier to get hold of a diet plan because trainers put together these programs keeping in mind the need of the dieter. Such a plan will have details like types of meals and snacks to take every day, the calories each has and the benefits that will result from the healthy foods.

On the other hand, if you want to lose weight on your own, the internet can be a great help. Ready-made diet plans are posted by coaches who help trainees via websites and discussion forums. Moreover, calorie counters are available on many websites that can be used to determine how many calories meals and snacks have.

The bottom line is that you have to burn more calories while exercising than the amount you consume. How many times have you felt a food temptation and thought, "It's okay, I can indulge- I just came from the gym...?" Thoughts like these are proof that dieters often overestimate the amount of calories they burn in a single workout session and eventually end up eating more than they actually did burn!

The next concern in regard to your diet, is that you may not be eating as healthy a one as you are supposed to. For instance, even if you have only one meal a day, if this meal is comprised of processed foods, your weight loss cycle will be completely unbalanced. Health is as important as eating little for obese people because the risk of many life threatening diseases comes in tow of being morbidly overweight.

Several studies in the United States have revealed that over the years the need for healthy eating has increased. However, people still don't necessarily eat healthy because the instances of heart diseases and Type 2 diabetes have gone up manifold in the last few years. The problem is, just like we tend to overestimate the calories we burn every day, we only *think* we eat healthy.

No one likes to admit how bad their diet is and so, each of us ends up thinking we're probably *not as bad as* the second person. Here's the black and white truth: when you make assumptions about how and what you are eating, you do not track the number of calories taken each day and hence, you never compare it to the cutoff you are actually supposed to be taking. Rings a bell?

With skewed dieting behaviors, neither the diet regime shows any results nor does your motivation to carry on diet lasts longer than a few weeks only. Nutritional research suggests that you always read labels of foods when purchasing them.

If you have been told to measure your portion sizes, please do so and always stick to the foods you are guided to eat. Foods such as chips, cakes, candies, packaged meat varieties, processed vegetables and deep fried, oily ingredients contain bad cholesterol, which is rich in heavy and addictive sugars as well as Omega 6 long chain fatty tissues that lead to the hundreds of diseases related to obesity.

On the other hand, freshly prepared homemade foods like pastas, omelets, steaks, boiled vegetables, baked seafood varieties, brown bread toasts and wheat cereals not only taste good, but are also diet friendly as well. Taking these makes you feel lighter, refreshed and up and running all day long!

2. Bad Habits That Hinder Weight Loss

Habits play a very important role in helping you lose weight. Healthy habits that make the body steer towards the right direction will urge you to stay away from indulgence and think clearly before you eat anything. In fact, if you ask an obese person why he can't control what he eats, the most likely answer will be, 'it's always been my habit.' Well, this habit isn't leading him anywhere, is it?

The reason diet plans and healthy regimes are called lifestyle choices is because they force the dieter to change his habits and adopt the ones that encourage healthy living. No matter which dieting regime you follow and no matter how many diets you have successfully completed- if you do not bring a positive change in your everyday behavior, all efforts go down the drain.

A very common habit among obese individuals is the lack of consistency. Such individuals will be ready to try new plans and weight loss regimes, but will never be consistent in what they begin. Moreover, as soon as the plan ends, all the restrain they had pulled up is directed towards celebratory eating. It is important to remember that diet plans teach a dieter consistency because even after the scheduled days of the plan are completed, the diet should become a way of life.

No one said no to an occasional indulgence; however, if the occasional indulgence because a religious ritual that is done thrice a week, the prospect of weight loss becomes pretty bleak, don't you think?

Another habit that is prized among weight loss circles is that of moderation. Moderation lies at the heart of any diet regime that promises to help you lose fat and give you a smart body. The essence of moderation is that you do not have to starve to death while dieting; instead, all you should strive for is a balanced meal plan.

Even if you find it hard to go through the day without the traditional three meals, that's really okay as long as you practice moderation. By eating smartly and being in control makes you alert and conscious of all that you are putting in your stomach. Portion control is also a part of moderation because it urges you to eat one serving of steak for dinner instead of the four that you would normally eat.

Moderation also applies to the frequency of 'treat' days you get. Like we discussed above, in a well-balanced diet plan, indulgence cannot be done thrice a week. Maybe thrice a month sounds more moderate?

We believe falling off the weight loss wagon is a natural setback for those trying really hard to shed extra pounds. But only if you are consistent will you be able to pull yourself back up. The more consistent and moderated you are in your habits, the better results you will see.

Lastly, habits that even the healthiest of the lot need to exercise control on is the urge to step on the weighing scale every two days. As a dieter, you have to understand that your body needs time to adapt to new changes. You didn't get obese in just a week did you? If you have spent a lifetime with bad eating habits, then at least give the body a month to show changes and record progress.

A majority of those who begin weight loss regimes are heard complaining often that the needle on the scale is not moving. There can be a lot of explanations for this. Firstly, if you are losing inches and your clothes are getting loose, you need not worry about the scales. As long as inches are cutting down, it is an indication that body fat is going down and is being replaced with hard muscles.

Secondly, you may be too frequent with stepping on the scales. Like we said, changes do not show in only a few days- which is why patience and consistency are keys to the success of a diet plan.

3. Exercises Routines

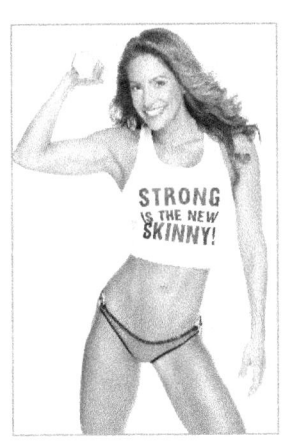

The third element of a successful weight loss regime is the exercise routines you are following. Exercising is a must- regardless of whether you need to shed a 100 pounds or merely 3 pounds to get back in shape. It is because of regular exercise that the body's physical activity levels increase which ultimately accelerate the fat burning cycle.

However, only knowing that you need to exercise in order to lose weight is only part of the information. The kind and type of exercise one does matters a lot too. When talked of in the context of weight loss, exercise takes a whole new meaning. Instead of just keeping you active, its aim becomes bringing a positive change to your physique.

In this regard, obese individuals are often recommended different types of exercises that target different areas of the body. For instance, if you are obese from the lower part of your body, exercises should aim to trim the thighs, sculpt the calves and tone the hips. If instead you carry on with very basic moves that do not target these areas, you are less likely to see results.

The second most important concern with exercising is whether you are relying *solely* on it for weight loss. If your plan is to lose weight by exercising and eating as you have always eaten, your plan will most definitely backfire. Why so? When you exercise, you will feel hungrier. Since you have placed no restraint on your eating habits, chances are that you will only end up eating more!

Yes, exercise does burn calories, but it takes a lot of time and effort to burn a very small amount of calories in an hour of exercise when you are panting and sweating. Even if you think you have done a lot, the truth of the matter is that only a couple of hundred calories are burnt with everyday exercising. For instance, it is known that intense exercise burns no more than 400-500 calories.

On the other hand, it often takes only 5 minutes to gobble down a thousand calories during the lunch break at work! Hence, if you rely on this trick alone, you are confronted with an uphill task. A combination of exercise and a healthy diet is what will bring the most change to your body.

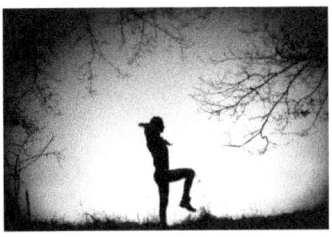

How Much Weight Can Get You In Trouble?

If your trainer asks you what did you eat today, how long does it take for you to think of an answer? If you have to rummage through your mind for 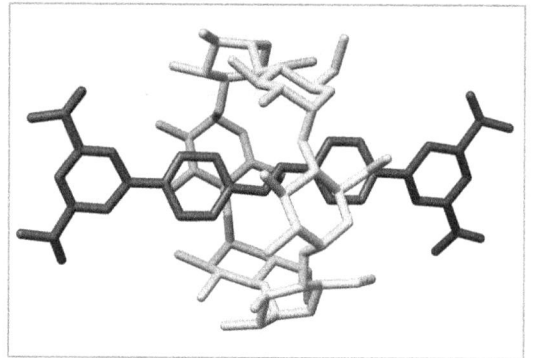 a few seconds, it is apparent that weight control is the least of your worries. Knowing what you ate and how much of it is an important indication of how healthy you are.

For many people, keeping a track of weight and eating habits is a waste of time. For them, the *real* work is to start exercising and cutting back on the foods they have heard are unhealthy. But wait a minute... how do you know how much weight you should be losing? How do you know what foods your body needs to stay away from? Do you even known what you weigh?

Being ignorant of the basics is the first wrong step in a series of many others, which often dictate the success or failure of a diet plan. Research has revealed that being organized while following a weight loss regime is the best way to make sure you see quick and fast results. This means no more running away from the dreaded task of weight watching!

The best way to do so is to keep a Food and Exercise Journal. Such a journal simply records everything you eat during a day, the exercise routine you complete, the general level of activity and the moods you go through. Recording these details has a very positive impact on a diet regime because it helps you stay on track. Every time you eat something that is unhealthy, it goes in the journal, making you extra cautious for the next time round.

Moreover, another benefit of keeping a journal is that it keeps tabs on your body weight before, during and after the diet regime. Now, we remember that in the last section we discussed the perils of relying on the scale way too much... but we 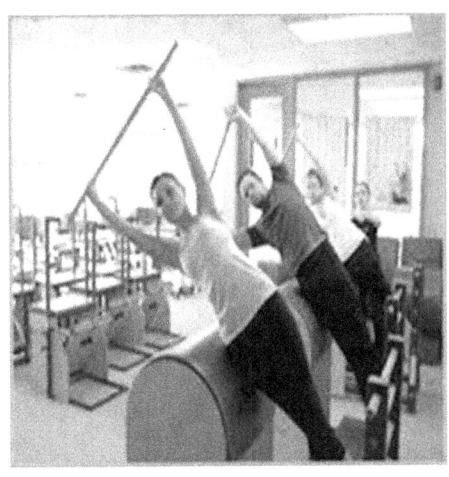 also discussed moderation, didn't we? While becoming obsessed about how much you weigh is wrong; not knowing what the ideal weight should be is even worse.

No two individuals have a similar body, and nor are they prone to change with the same stimuli. According to this notion, the ideal weight for every body type is different and it takes a whole new approach for two people to achieve the same ideal weight. Hence, the first step is to know what you weigh and where you should be to become ideal.

Body Mass Index

What Is BMI?

The foundation of every diet regime lies in the Body Mass Index of an individual. Depending on how much a person weighs, a diet plan that highlights the needs of the body can be customized and tailor made to suit this particular 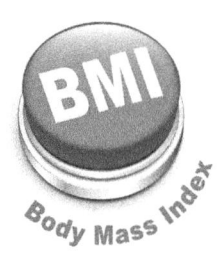 individual. Despite being aware of the hundreds of fancy diet fads on the internet, an average person trying to lose weight may still be unaware of what the BMI is and its importance in maintaining a healthy body.

The BMI is a measure that compares the relative weight of an individual with two attributes, namely, the mass and height. BMI is a standard that is used widely in calculations of ideal weights for people who have different heights and amounts of mass in their body. Over the years, the various

BMI values have been arranged in the form of a table for easy reference.

In the early years of its development, this index was only used for research and studies conducted on sizable populations. However, as obesity became an immediate problem in the western societies, the popularity of BMI soared as an index that could put together three important components which were essential in determining the health of a person.

The main aim for BMI has always been to give an idea of how much an individual should weigh and what levels of activity he should indulge in. However, treating it as an end in itself is not the right approach.

How To Measure BMI?

To make the calculation of BMI easier, the following formula is used as a metric:

$$BMI = \frac{mass(kg)}{(height(m))^2} \quad OR \quad = \frac{mass(lb)}{(height(in))^2} \times 703$$

According to this formula, BMI is proportional to the mass of a person and inversely proportional to his height. This means, as height increases, the Body Mass Index decreases. For instance, if a person weighs 130 pounds and is 5 feet 6 inches tall, he would have a BMI of 20.5.

BMI is a straight forward and simple calculation with this formula, which is why it is being used today as a preliminary assessment of overweight individuals who want start effective weight loss programs. The biggest use of this metric comes when a nutritionist assesses whether a dieter needs to lose weight or not.

BMI is listed as a relative value for every height and weight category. When the nutritionist matches your current weight with the current height, you can fall into a number of classifications that are called BMI Standards. Depending on the particular standard of your height and weight, you will be advised to lose or gain weight respectively.

BMI Standards

BMI Standards are very important, because on its own, a BMI of 10, 20or 30 has no value. If a doctor tells you your BMI is 18, how do you know if you are healthy 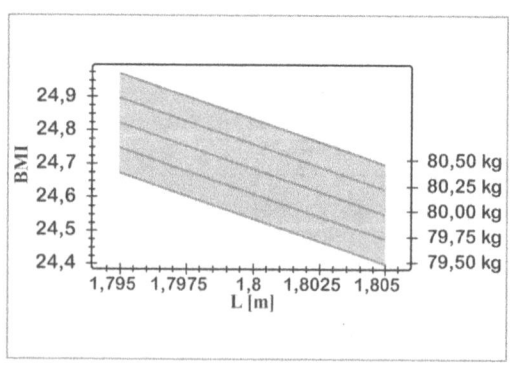 or not? For this figure to make sense and to help draw a conclusion, it has to be compared to certain standards that have been established by health care professionals and experts.

While a thin person may be classified as very thin by some and moderately thin by others; for the sake of standardization, five main weight categories are defined for the BMI Standards. These classifications are universally acceptable, although some variations exist in each depending on the country you live in.

- Underweight: Individuals are classified as Underweight if their BMI is less than 18.5. These people are told to gain weight to become healthy.

- Healthy Weight: Individuals are classified as Healthy if their BMI is within the range of 18.5 to 25. Such individuals are told to maintain weight to prevent health risks.

- Overweight: Individuals are classified as Overweight if their BMI is between 25 and 30. Being slightly overweight, these individuals may be asked to lose a few pounds to become healthy.

- Obese: Individuals are classified as Obese if their BMI is between 30 and 40. Losing weight for these individuals is a must.

- Morbidly Obese: Individuals are classified as Morbidly Obese if their BMI is over 40. Morbidly obese people are at a high risk of losing their life if their weight does not decrease gradually. Moreover, their body conditions are deemed highly sensitive- so much so that a sudden drop in weight may also be dangerous.

Based on these classifications, medical professionals are able to detect early signs of potential diseases and ailments as well. For instance, people who have a BMI of over 40 are at a high risk of Type 2 Diabetes, Heart attack and Colorectal Cancer- all of which are near fatal illnesses that can rob the patient of a good life. Spotting these conditions early on- before the symptoms start to manifest themselves- is a very useful way to steer people towards healthy living and urging them to lose weight that is enough to guarantee a reduction in the risk of these diseases.

Similarly, a BMI that classifies an individual as Underweight is not healthy either. Even though it suggests that the person is not fat or at the risk of diseases that are related to obesity, it points out that the body may not be receiving adequate nutrition. Anemia is one of the most common health conditions that many people face in their teens and adult years.

Being underweight on the BMI Scale also suggests that you may be prone to a high risk of Osteoporosis, which is the gradual weakening and erosion of bones. Osteoporosis has no definite cure. It can be curbed by healthy intake of foods and liquids. However, when malnutrition turns into this problem, preventing bone weakness is not all that easy.

BMI Comparison Chart

To make BMI comparison and reference a piece of cake, experts have put together a chart that makes it very easy for dieters and non-dieters to check their BMI score and determine how healthy they are. This chart has all the

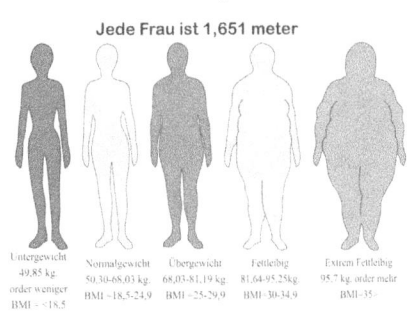

calculations done for you, along with BMI classifications written at the top, so that you do not have to go through the tedious data collection and calculation process.

With this chart, all you have to do is spot the weight range you belong to and read the corresponding height in inches. Next, see the BMI classification to which this weight and height belong. Different charts have been made with different perspectives in mind. Sometimes, the charts being used are color coded to make it easy for people to quickly refer to the BMI classification they should be concerned with.

The following is one such table that can easily be read by anyone trying to see how healthy his body is. This particular table is very comprehensive because it gives the weight in both, Kilograms and Pounds and the height in both Inches and Centimeters. See the five different colors in the chart? Each represents a category of the BMI classification.

Gewicht lbs	100	105	110	115	120	125	130	135	140	145	150	155	160	165	170	175	180	185	190	195	200	205	210	215
kg	45,5	47,7	50,0	52,3	54,5	55,8	59,1	61,4	63,6	65,9	68,2	70,5	72,7	75,0	77,3	79,5	81,8	84,1	86,4	88,6	90,9	93,2	95,5	97,7

Höhe in/cm — Untergewicht | Gesund | Übergewicht | Fettleibig | Extrem Fettleibig

Höhe in/cm	100	105	110	115	120	125	130	135	140	145	150	155	160	165	170	175	180	185	190	195	200	205	210	215
5'00" - 152,4	19	20	21	22	23	24	25	26	27	28	29	30	31	32	33	34	35	36	37	38	39	40	41	42
5'01" - 154,9	18	19	20	21	22	23	24	25	26	27	28	29	30	31	32	33	34	35	36	36	37	38	39	40
5'02" - 157,4	18	19	20	21	22	22	23	24	25	26	27	28	29	30	31	32	33	33	34	35	36	37	38	39
5'03" - 160,0	17	18	19	20	21	22	23	24	24	25	26	27	28	29	30	31	32	32	33	34	35	36	37	38
5'04" - 162,5	17	18	18	19	20	21	22	23	24	24	25	26	27	28	29	30	31	31	32	33	34	35	36	37
5'05" - 165,1	16	17	18	19	20	20	21	22	23	24	25	25	26	27	28	29	30	30	31	32	33	34	35	35
5'06" - 167,6	16	17	17	18	19	20	21	21	22	23	24	25	25	26	27	28	29	29	30	31	32	33	34	34
5'07" - 170,1	15	16	17	18	18	19	20	21	22	22	23	24	25	25	26	27	28	29	29	30	31	32	33	33
5'08" - 172,7	15	16	16	17	18	19	19	20	21	22	22	23	24	25	25	26	27	28	28	29	30	31	32	32
5'09" - 175,2	14	15	16	17	17	18	19	20	20	21	22	22	23	24	25	25	26	27	26	28	25	30	31	31
5'10" - 177,8	14	15	15	16	17	18	18	19	20	20	21	22	22	23	24	25	25	26	27	28	26	29	30	30
5'11" - 180,3	14	14	15	16	16	17	18	18	19	20	21	31	22	23	23	24	25	25	26	27	27	28	29	30
6'00" - 182,8	13	14	14	15	16	17	17	18	19	19	20	21	21	22	23	23	24	25	25	26	27	27	28	29
6'01" - 185,4	13	13	14	15	15	16	17	17	18	19	19	20	21	21	22	23	23	24	25	25	26	27	27	28
6'02" - 187,9	12	13	14	14	15	16	16	17	18	18	19	19	20	21	21	22	23	23	24	25	25	26	27	27
6'03" - 190,5	12	13	13	14	15	15	16	16	17	18	18	19	20	20	21	21	22	23	23	24	25	25	26	26
6'04" - 193,0	12	12	13	14	14	15	15	16	17	17	18	18	19	20	20	21	22	22	23	23	24	25	25	26

For instance, if you weigh 150 pounds and your height is 5'04, your BMI turns out to be 25. The area in which 25 lies is colored yellow; and according to the key at the top yellow represents Overweight. Hence, with this weight and height your body is slightly overweight for which you should contact a health care specialist to get hold of a diet plan.

Limitations of BMI

Even though BMI has gained tremendous importance as a measure of how healthy an individual is, there is a lot of stir in health circles regarding the limitations of this metric. At first, when the Body Mass Index was developed, health experts and doctors considered it to be *the* ideal standard for body mass classifications.

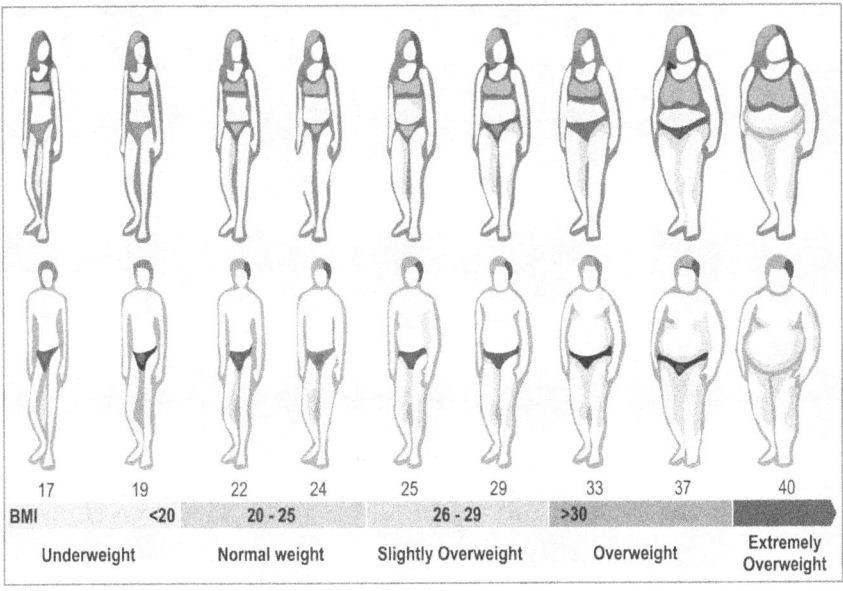

However, soon enough, the many shortcomings of this approach surfaced. This isn't to say that the BMI is wrong, or that it is not a credible measure of the idea weight one should be at. Instead, it suffices to say that even when BMI is used, a lot of other biological, social and psychological factors should be taken into account to make sure that the weight analysis is complete and comprehensive.

The following are some limitations of the Body Mass Index:

- Even though BMI takes into account the mass, height and weight of a person, it fails to account for the fact that these three quantities do not always increase proportionately. A very tall person may be too thin or too fat and a very short person may be too fat or too thin. There can be any number of combinations, thus treating BMI as a last resort is not sensible.

- BMI is a widely used approach because it presents a standard. However, it should be known that there is an element of subjectivity inherent in this approach to healthy weight classification. Depending on various countries and their health standards, BMI classifications differ. For instance, till 1998, the healthy weight limit in the United States was 27. From this year onwards, the country started following the limits set by the World Health Organization (18.5- 25), turning 25 million people overweight in just one day!

- Similarly, before 1998, the same person with a BMI of 26.8 would have been healthy in the United States and Obese in Japan.

- BMI ignores the part played by gender differences. For instance, it has been proven by research that women have an added layer of fat that men don't. Taking this into account, does it mean more women are unhealthy and more men are healthy?

- Similarly, BMI leaves out age classifications as well. Older people tend to have a higher fat percentage than younger people. Would a similar BMI point out this difference?

- BMI, an important metric that it is, also doesn't take into account bone mass and muscle density. For individuals with a higher muscle density, the BMI will be very high; however, it does not necessarily mean they are unhealthy. Athletes who have a very high percentage of muscle and a very low percentage of fat always have a very high BMI because most of their weight lies in the muscle fibers.

- The BMI also does not specify the body type you have. Determining whether you are pear or apple shaped is important in the context of medicine because the location of fat plays a huge role in keeping you healthy. Hence, when it comes to the body type, BMI gives the incomplete picture.

- BMI does not always represent changes in lifestyle. For instance, say you have a healthy BMI, but you tend to stay inactive when it comes to physical effort. When you incorporate exercise into your daily routine, this positive change in lifestyle will not be recorded by BMI- meaning you will still be classified in the same category as you were previously.

- Lastly, just like age and gender, BMI doesn't take into account ethnicity, which has a huge impact on health and heredity diseases. For instance, it is a known fact that Asian-Americans are more prone to heart attacks, even at a lower BMI, than Native Americans. Hence, for Asians the obesity cutoff begins at 27 instead of the standard of 30.

Healthy Weight Chart

From all the discussion above, it should now be clear to you that the importance of being within a healthy weight range cannot be put into words. Obesity is one of the most dangerous health conditions that often top diseases like AIDS and Breast Cancer. For some, having a healthy weight is not hard because obesity is not in their genes; while for others it may be synonymous to going to the moon and back!

As discussed previously, there are a lot of reasons that can lead to weight gain, some which are not in the control of the individual at all. Eating disorders and ailments that add extra pounds can be hard to fight because they present a problem that cannot be curbed by simply emptying your refrigerator one fine day. However, despite the reasons, a lot of effort needs to be put into becoming healthy by one and all if the quality of life is to be maintained.

A lot of research in nutritional circles reveals that weight differences are highly dependent on gender. Both men and women have different daily requirements for food because their bodies work very differently. The most predominant reason for these differences is the presence of various hormones in men and women that regulate the functioning of the body.

Broadly speaking, women are known to have more fat content than men. An average woman has 25% of fat, while an average man has 15% fat in his body. Owing to these differences, women require fewer calories per day to reach a healthy meal cut off than men do. The most common reason for these differences is that since women have to carry a fetus at some point in their lives, this extra layer of fat ensures safety and a regular supply of energy.

For this reason, any health standardization that is made across genders is not representative of these differences, which is why it may be misleading or give only part of the information needed to determine the ideal weight standards.

The BMI calculations are scrutinized for similar reasons. As mentioned previously, experts believe that the biggest reason BMI fails to be a comprehensive metric is because it does not take into account factors like age that matter a lot in the discussion of healthy weight.

The following is a table that explains in detail, the weight ranges that are classified as healthy for women. Take a look at Table 2 that gives the same information for men. There is a marked difference between the ranges for men and women, and now you know why!

Table 3 on the following page gives the healthy weight ranges for children. Even though weight loss becomes a fashion and aesthetic concern for individuals once they mature, parents should nonetheless keep tabs on how healthy their child is It is a well-known fact that the eating habits that children develop in the initial years are carried on the teens and adult years as well.

Letting a child munch on unhealthy snacks from an early age conditions his or her mind to believe that these snacks are good for health. Moreover, it makes children overweight in their own age brackets. According to a research from 1980 to 2012, the number of obese children increased by 18% in the United States.

When obesity grips a child at a very young age, it is even harder to lose weight and become fit. Since the excess fat in a child's body turns from soft to hard over the passage of years , it is usually too late by the time he realizes that he is overweight by social standards. From that point onwards, the road to becoming healthy is marred with a lot of psychological pressures. At this point, the chances of developing eating disorders and becoming a victim to ailments like high blood pressure and premature Diabetes increase tremendously.

Childhood obesity has become a top concern for health practitioners in the United States. With children being conditioned to eat fast-food and unhealthy snacks from a young age, doctors and nutritionists worry that the onset of child diabetes and cancer will become a definite occurrence. The possible solution? Educating children on the benefits of eating a healthy diet.

Table 1- Healthy Weight Table for Women Aged Between 25 to 59 Years

Height in Feet&Inches	Small Frame	Medium Frame	Large Frame
4'10"	102 - 111	109 - 121	118-131
4'11"	103 - 113	111 - 123	120-134
5'0"	104 - 115	113 - 126	122-137
5'1"	106 - 118	115 - 129	125-140
5'2"	108 - 121	118 - 132	128-143
5'3"	111 - 124	121 - 135	131-147
5'4"	114 - 127	124 - 138	134-151
5'5"	117 - 130	127 - 141	137-155
5'6"	120 - 133	130 - 144	140-159
5'7"	123 - 136	133 - 147	143-163
5'8"	126 - 139	136 - 150	146-167
5'9"	129 - 142	139 - 153	149-170
5'10"	132 - 145	142 - 156	152-173
5'11"	135 - 148	145 - 159	155-176
6'0"	138 - 151	148 - 162	158-179

Table 2- Healthy Weight Table for Men Aged Between 25 to 59 Years

Height in Feet&Inches	Small Frame	Medium Frame	Large Frame
5'2"	128 - 134	131 - 141	138 - 150
5'3"	130 - 136	133 - 143	140 - 153
5'4"	132 - 138	135 - 145	142 - 156
5'5"	134 - 140	137 - 148	144 - 160
5'6"	136 - 142	139 - 151	146 - 164
5'7"	138 - 145	142 - 154	149 - 168
5'8"	140 - 148	145 - 157	152 - 172
5'9"	142 - 151	151 - 163	155 - 176
5'10"	144 - 154	151 - 163	158 - 180
5'11"	146 - 157	154 - 166	161 - 184
6'0"	149 - 160	157 - 170	164 - 188
6'1"	152 - 164	160 - 174	168 - 192
6'2"	155 - 168	165 - 178	172 - 197
6'3"	158 - 172	167 - 182	176 - 202
6'4"	162 - 176	171 - 187	181 - 207

Table 3- Healthy Weight Ranges for Girls and Boys

BOYS		GIRLS	
Age 1 year	21- 26 pounds	Age 1 year	17- 24 pounds
Age 2 years	23- 32 pounds	Age 2 years	22- 31 pounds
Age 3 years	27- 37 pounds	Age 3 years	26- 36 pounds
Age 4 years	30- 42 pounds	Age 4 years	29- 41 pounds
Age 5 years	34- 50 pounds	Age 5 years	33- 48 pounds
Age 6 years	39- 56 pounds	Age 6 years	37- 56 pounds
Age 7 years	43- 65 pounds	Age 7 years	41- 64 pounds
Age 8 years	48- 72 pounds	Age 8 years	53- 73 pounds
Age 9 years	53- 80 pounds	Age 9 years	49- 84 pounds
Age 10 years	57- 92 pounds	Age 10 years	53- 96 pounds
Age 11 years	62- 105 pounds	Age 11 years	58- 116 pounds
Age 12 years	67- 119 pounds	Age 12 years	64- 124 pounds
Age 13 years	72- 134 pounds	Age 13 years	72- 134 pounds
Age 14 years	80- 147 pounds	Age 14 years	83- 144 pounds
Age 15 years	91- 160 pounds	Age 15 years	89- 151 pounds
Age 16 years	103- 172 pounds	Age 16 years	92- 155 pounds
Age 17 years	111- 182 pounds	Age 17 years	94- 158 pounds
Age 18 years	114- 188 pounds	Age 18 years	98- 160 pounds

The Game Plan

How to Lose Weight without Sacrificing Your Diet

So, what's the game plan? How should you start losing weight after you see the warning signs as you fall in the yellow colored region of the BMI table? We have referred to weight loss and dieting regimes as a complete change in lifestyle because these plans have to be incorporated into a person's daily routine.

If you think you can get rid of the tons of extra fat layers by treating a diet as a short term inclusion, you will be disappointed as the prescribed three month period comes to a close. It is for this reason that the game plan for weight loss is nothing less than a New Plan to Live!

Unfortunately, there is a lot of confusion when it comes to losing weight. There are millions of diet and exercise plans on the internet and in hard copies of famous books- all of which assert a different option. Readers are often lost on how to begin any diet plan at all because they find themselves unable to pick and choose which ones will be most beneficial.

While each of these plans would have been formulated by knowledgeable experts; if it is hard to follow and maintain, it is not worthy of being chosen. Remember, the beauty of a diet regime lies in its simplicity. Losing weight shouldn't be made hard because it requires a lot of effort and self-restraint as it is. If dieters are made to choose and assess the efficacy of complicated regimes, the entire purpose of returning-to-the-basics with healthy food will be lost completely.

Therefore, whenever you want to decide how to put a stop to the life of unhealthy eating habits; all you need to do is befriend your body again and go back to the basics. It is as simple as that.

Are Healthy Bodies Made In The Kitchen?

In regards to weight loss, many people often ask the question, 'What's more important, diet or exercise?' To a health enthusiast, these people may come off as lazy and simply not interested in getting healthy. Why wouldn't you do both, exercise and diet? In the previous sections, we have asserted time and again that the importance of a complete and comprehensive weight loss program can never be underestimated.

Only when a weight loss regime targets all possible aspects, does it become effective. However, growing concern about obesity and the efficacy of fancy diets has led many people to repeat the same question again and again. As hard as it may be to believe, there is some hidden truth in the statement that 'healthy bodies are made in the kitchen'.

- **Eating Healthy**

According to Shawn M. Talbott, a Nutritional Biochemist, healthy eating makes up for 75% of a weight loss regime, with the remaining 25% allotted to exercise. For Talbott, the merits of eating healthy can be complimented with exercise, but can never be outweighed. Several studies have been conducted in the last few years to confirm this hypothesis.

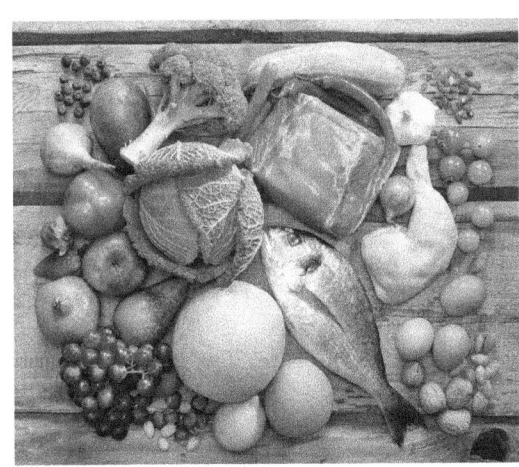

In one particular study, dieters were divided into two groups. One group was told to exercise and the other was told to diet only for a period of 15 weeks. After this duration, individuals in the second group that aimed to lose weight with diet alone lost 23 pounds, while those belonging to the first group, lost only 6 pounds.

The rationale behind this conclusion, according to Talbott, is that it is always easier to lose weight by avoiding/cutting the calorie intake; instead of eating calories and then burning them off later. This conclusion is coherent with our analysis in the above chapters because we concluded that most dieters always overestimate the number of calories they have burned during one workout session. Let's take an example. If you avoid eating a scrumptious, yet overly filling Quesadilla meal, you can avoid putting in 500+ calories in your system; OR you can run 4 miles the next day to burn these calories off!

The best way to keep an eye out for healthy eating is to set a mark, i.e. 10 calories per pound of body weight. So if you weigh 140 pounds, your intake should be limited to 1400 calories on a daily basis. Anything more will be excess-hindering the fat burning cycle- and anything less will result in a very slow and sluggish metabolism that is again not an ideal situation for weight loss.

Therefore, managing a healthy diet is the biggest secret to losing weight and if done properly, you should be able to see results regardless of how long you exercise for.

- **Hitting The Gym**

Michele Olson, PhD and Professor of Physical Education at the University Of Montgomery, Alabama,

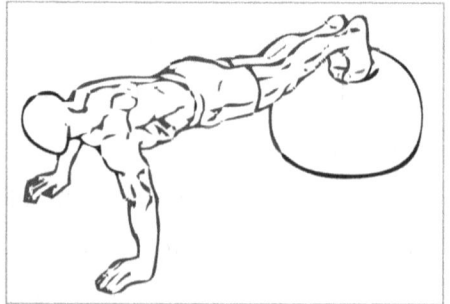

agrees with Talbott that weight loss can be spurred by a healthy diet alone. However, being well versed with the importance of physical activity, Olson says that for the short-term weight loss to be sustained and accelerated in the long term, exercise should be made part of the process.

Without adequate exercise, dieters lose only a portion of fat that has bulked up in the body; the rest of lose comes from the weakening of muscles and a decrease in bone density. It is only when the dieters start to work out, do they build muscle fiber and stimulate the growth of muscle tissues in the right parts of the body.

Moreover, these exercises do not have to be very hard either. The easiest way to complement a healthy diet with exercise is to begin a Cardio Program that leads to rapid fat burning. Similarly, a couple of Zumba moves the next day and a few hours of brisk walking and jogging on another, and you are all set on the path to successful weight loss.

Oh, and not to forget the other positive effects of exercise on the overall quality of life like better mental strength, lower stress levels and an improved sleep cycle. With these benefits in tow, exercise should definitely be on your agenda; even if it comes second to dieting.

The Verdict?

No matter how much weight you need to shed or how fast; a bad diet can never be fixed with any power on the face of the planet. A great exercise plan cannot undo the negative effects of a diet that robs the dieter of healthy nutrition and instead gives him problems such as bad fats and lipids. Hence, if you absolutely must put diet on one scale and exercise on the other, the one with diet will weigh heavier.

This isn't to say that exercise should be an option when you try to lose weight. Exercising is an essential cog in this entire equation. However, when it comes to placing them along a scale of importance, diet comes before exercise because only a healthy diet can help you exercise better.

The Weight Loss Weapon

Now that we have established that the weight loss cycle pivots more towards a healthy diet than it does towards exercise alone, it is easy to point out the things that 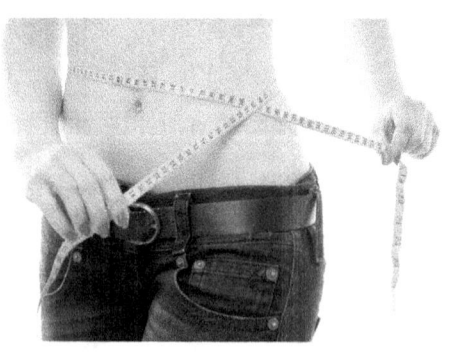 you absolutely must do and those that you can keep on the sides. Remember, exercise is important because it builds muscles that occupy less space in the body; it is by no means unnecessary.

However, the type, hours and timings of exercises can be managed and tweaked to your comfort when you are following a diet plan that is at par with the amount of calories you should be consuming. If you wanted one weapon that could lead you through the entire weight loss process, would you jump at the opportunity?

For modern weight loss gurus, this weapon is the Protein in our food. For decades, a major misconception has been tied to protein rich foods. People believe that these foods, while give an approved quantity of protein, are very high in calories too. Hence, instead of having a sizable serving of pan grilled steak, dieters preferred having a plain slice of bread.

Busting this myth has led to the resurfacing of the low-carb diet. Experts suggest that foods that are rich in carbohydrates are the ones to avoid because they give the dieter a heavy and fulfilled feeling. In fact, the lower belly 'pooch' that most of us find annoying is also attributed to heavy carbohydrate intake.

This notion by diet planning specialists and trainers has been further confirmed by nutritionists as well who are now concerned about the staggeringly low protein count in the most common foods consumed today. Most women between 20 and 40 years of age do not receive the average dose of protein they should be taking for a healthy lifestyle.

This macro-nutrient that makes up the biggest chunk of our muscles is one of the most important ingredients to be consumed on a daily basis, especially if you are gunning to lose weight. Moreover, proteins are broken down into amino acids by the body- these substances are in high demand when you replenish your system after an intense workout regime.

Protein Power

The rationale behind this claim is simple. When you work-out to lose weight, you burn calories and also begin a process called Muscle Breakdown. While the calorie 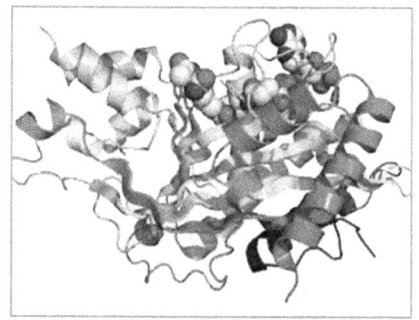 burning process is great; the latter is not because by losing muscle, your body fails to achieve the lean and trimmed look you desire.

Using the amino acids that you consume with protein rich foods, the body is able to synthesize lean muscles that have the power to speed up the metabolic system. And what's the result? With strong muscle fibers, you lose calories faster even when you are not exercising because the body is geared towards protein buildup.

This is the reason that once you are in full shape after months of effort and patience, a cookie here and there does not affect your physique because the accelerated metabolic cycle is adept at burning calories faster than ever before. Hence, instead of bulking up and increasing the percentage of fat, proteins aim to increase the percentage of muscle. This way, you lose weight, but unnecessary muscle breakdown does not happen, which leads to a well-toned and smart body.

Moreover, protein rich foods require a lot of energy to be digested and broken down. When you eat a healthy lunch of seafood and vegetables, your body needs a lot of energy to break down the proteins and use them for muscle building. But where does it get this energy? You guessed it; it burns more calories that are already present in the system to get enough energy to process a protein rich diet.

Once processed, proteins also curb hunger by leaving the stomach at a very slow pace. For a dieter who is watching his weight, this translates into a fuller stomach and an urge to go without more food for longer. This hypothesis was proved by a study that was conducted for a 12 week period. During this time, dieters were divided into two groups; one that was told to take 30% more protein and the other one acting as a control.

With this change in diet, the group the consumed more protein ate 450 calories less every day and lost 11 pounds in total without any other changes to their diet.

How Much Protein Is Enough?

So, how much protein should you be taking? When will you know if it's enough? According to experts, 0.5 grams to 1 gram of protein per pound of body weight is enough for an adult. This means, if you weigh 140 pounds,

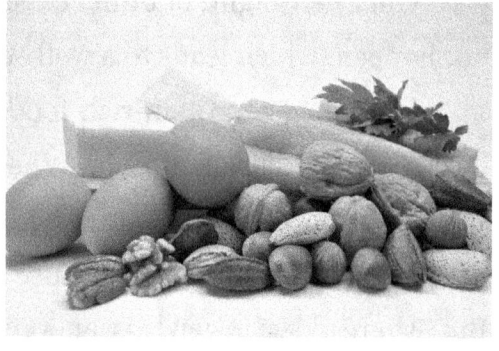

your protein requirement is between 70 grams to 140 grams. Making sure your intake is actually somewhere between these limits, we recommend you keep a rough count of the number of proteins in the most common foods you eat.

Moreover, nutritionists suggest that at least 30 grams from the 70-140grams range should be consumed in the morning. When you wake up on an empty stomach, proteins can come to the rescue if you consume foods like eggs, sausages and fresh fruits. A protein rich breakfast keeps the body going for longer because it feels satiated and is ready to take up the hectic responsibilities of the day ahead.

However, here's a catch. Not all protein sources contain the nine amino acids that are necessary for the body. Some foods that have protein are incomplete sources, and hence are not enough for daily consumption alone. To be precise, animal proteins contain the complete set of proteins that are needed by the body for useful protein synthesis.

Foods to incorporate in your diet include; seafood varieties, chicken, turkey, pork, lean beef and low fat dairy items.

5 Foods That Do The Work For You

Another myth tied to healthy eating for weight loss is that no matter how much a dieter tries, healthy food can never be made tasty. Not only is 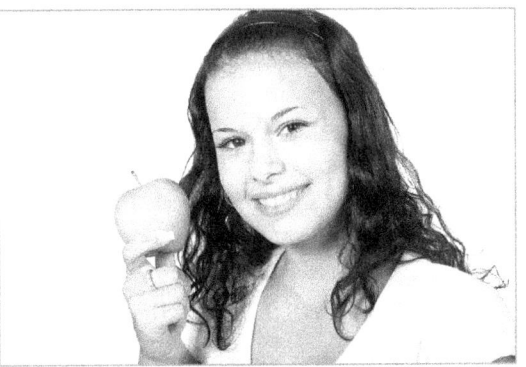 this notion deeply rooted, it has become one of the biggest obstacles dieters face when trying to lose weight because they feel everything they will directed to eat will taste bad and be like a pill they have to swallow hard.

If you are one of these people, you couldn't be more mistaken. Healthy eating can very well be delicious. In fact, the more heart you put into the diet regime, the better you will be able to think of low calorie dishes that are great for the taste palette as well. Moreover, apart from full course meals, a lot of healthy snacks can be on a dieter's radar because they help curb hunger and have a very positive impact on weight loss.

In short, they do all the work for you!

1. Apples: A medium Apple contains only 95 calories and is packed with loads of fiber and varying quantities of vitamin C and Potassium. Fiber intake is essential for those aiming for weight loss because it helps regulate bowel movements to encourage the passage of waste, thus improving the overall health of a dieter.

2. Soups: Soups are a delicious alternative to heavy meals because they curb hunger for hours. Moreover, when taken with a meal, research proves that people who begin with a delicious bowl of soup end up eating 20% fewer calories.

3. Sweet Potatoes: Baked sweet potatoes have as few as 100 calories. These foods make for amazing and super yummy appetizers and sidelines with soups and salads.

Moreover, it is a powerhouse for fiber, potassium, vitamin C, magnesium, iron and 438% of vitamin A that is responsible for healthy eyesight.

4. Raspberries: Raspberries are one of those delicious berries that have a lot of fiber and are very low in calories. Not only do they lower cholesterol, they work like magic for cutting down on belly fat.

5. Chickpeas: Chickpeas are widely used in salads and spicy snacks because they have a natural flavor of their own. A 3/4th cup of Chickpeas has 8 grams of fiber and Vitamin B6, which is essential for the manufacture of new cells and muscles. Make sure to include this bean in your diet at least once a week.

The Million Dollar Diet Plan

What then makes up for a million dollar diet plan? Is it something so out of the world that most of us haven't been able to benefit from it? Or is this plan so overtly simple

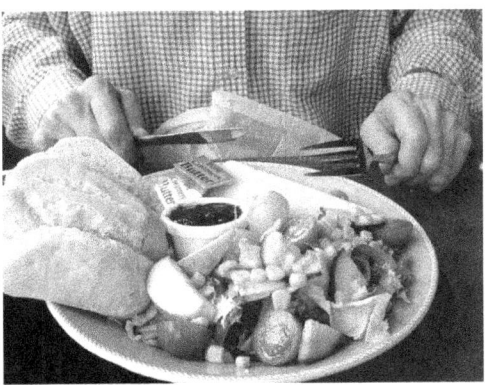

that we fail to acknowledge it at all? There is a lot that one needs to know about the perfect diet plan... beginning with the news that there is no such thing as perfect!

The Million Dollar Diet Plan is not literally worth millions of dollars; in fact, it is worth way more in terms of its simplicity, adaptability and efficacy. While you wouldn't have to spend all this money to make sure you set foot on the right track to weight loss.

The most important thing to remember about a diet plan is that the best plan differs from one person to the other. For someone who has to lose a 100 pounds, a different diet plan will have to be tailored from scratch, while for another person who merely needs to shed 10 pounds to get back in shape, the diet plan will be starkly different.

This said, there are a number of aspects of a weight loss plan that do remain the same across the board. These are, perhaps, the few elements that make a plan worth a million dollars- or worth nothing at all. The purpose of this book is to help you grasp these essentials without making you spend thousands of dollars on diet books and paid plans that may or may not work.

The perfect diet plan has the following at its heart:

I. A regular cardio plan that is carried out at a fixed time of the day. This cardio plan should be considered very important because it tones the body and helps it replace fat with muscle.

II. A consistent and healthy eating schedule. Such a schedule may look like this:

1) Breakfast

- One cup black tea/coffee
- 2 hard-boiled eggs or scrambled eggs

2) Lunch

- One portion of chicken fillet seasoned and pan grilled
- Sautéed vegetables on the side
- One glass lemon flavored water

3) Evening Snack

- One apple OR 4-5 almonds OR 4-5 Raspberries

4) Dinner

- A bowl of seasoned vegetable soup with a piece of bread
- Grilled fish
- A cup of Ginger Tea (2-3 hours after dinner)

III. A healthy sleeping pattern. Getting at least 6-7 hours of sleep is essential for those hoping to lose fat with a diet regime because lack of sleep is one of the biggest de-motivators to staying healthy. If you are cranky and sleepy all day, would you care what you eat? We don't think so!

IV.   Healthy habits and personality traits. As discussed previously, the kind of everyday habits you have play a huge role in determining how successful a diet plan will be. Being patient, consistent, dedicated and forward looking are a few personality traits that make all the difference in this regard.

Do I Have to Run 3 Miles?

This depends on whether you want to lose those extra pounds or not. People who want to achieve their dream and ideal weight but do not want to exercise or work 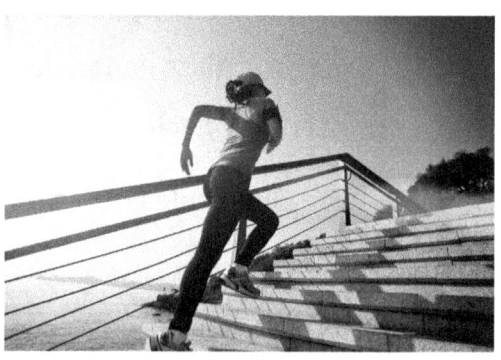 hard for it can easily be likened to people who wish to earn loads of money without having to go to work. Nothing in this world worth having comes without any amount of effort, and the same goes for a good toned figure. You cannot lose weight without having to work for it, which is why, you would have to exercise and control your diet if you wish to look good.

Exercises that Work

The types of exercises that are bound to work for you mainly depend upon the type of body shape you have. If you have an apple shape, a pear shape, and so on, then your exercise regimen is going to vary according to those particular details. However, there are still a few basic good exercises that you can apply in your day to day lifestyle to make you thin and fit. These exercises are something that you can learn to incorporate in your life slowly and steadily so that you can build your stamina overtime and maintain it instead of giving it your all the first week around but then giving up the second week because it was a little too tough to maintain for you.

These exercises may seem a little tough to you but bear it in mind that these exercises work a great deal and they are super effective when it comes to losing weight and keeping it off. Listed below are a few different types of exercises that you should most definitely incorporate in your day to day lifestyle so that you never have to complain about not fitting into that dress you fancy any longer:

1. Push ups

Push up seem to be very a very difficult type of exercise however when it comes to effectiveness, these one come at first place and there is most definitely a profound reason for that. Pushups may seem like an exercise that only engage your upper 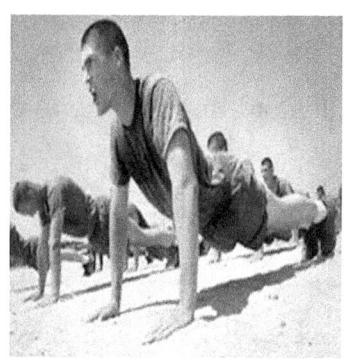 body but the truth is that they engage your entire body, but most importantly, they engage the core of the body which is essential in giving you the inner strength to continue on with the exercise and allows you to lose weight in a significantly short time.

Whenever you are doing your pushups and find yourself not able to continue any longer, try to concentrate all your energy on your core which is in the center of your body. Consider it to be that one point and center of gravity from which all of your strength resonates throughout your entire body. This is the place all your muscles derive their strength from and this is the place that enables you to carry on even when you cannot muster up the energy to do so.

When you start doing pushups, please do not start with 20 pushups because this is an unrealistic target; one that no matter what happens, you will never be able to achieve on the very first day. Set your maximum target to seven pushups first in the first two weeks of your exercise program, and then move on to other types of exercises. If you find that you still cannot do seven pushups in the military style then there is a solution for that too. You can place your knees on the ground and just lift your upper body instead. These types of pushups will be easier than the military style pushups and can prove to be good baby steps towards building your stamina for more.

When two weeks have passed, your muscles have gone past their sore quality and you find it easier to life yourself up, try to add two or three more to the regimen but if you have been doing the pushups with your knees on the ground then try to do the additional two or three pushups in the military style exercise. This is so that your strength for that particular ability also builds up and so that your body also gets used to it in a better and safer way than exerting yourself and scaring yourself away from the mere concept and idea of exercise.

Always remember the fact that pushups may seem difficult and they may not make you feel so pleasant but in due time they have the capability to make you lose weight and to make you look amazing. Pushups tone your upper muscles in a way that no other exercise can, which is why even if you are a woman and cannot muster up enough strength, then work up to it. Do as many as you feel comfortable with and then start adding a small number every two weeks to get to your target pushup number.

2. Jogging or Running

You may have already heard it but jogging and running are probably two of the best exercises to not only stay slim but also to stay fit. This is because this is a great 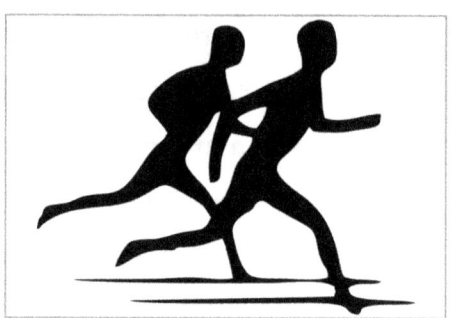 cardio exercise and can not only tone your body and your muscles but it also caters to the organs inside of your body. Your heart, lungs, and even areas such as your skin can look wondrous when you start running or jogging particularity in the morning. The earlier you start developing this habit the better it is going to be for you.

When you jog you not only engage your core and derive energy from it but you also tone your muscles in a way that makes them supple and smooth. Your skin remains hydrated which means that you stay away from things such as acne and other skin problems. Your leg muscles, which are the hardest to get into shape, become smooth and toned in a matter of a few weeks.

Jogging and running also greatly reduce stress levels which automatically decrease your food intake. Even if you are not a stress eater, you still opt for unhealthier food when you are upset as opposed to healthy food. When you are upset or stressed you do not feel like eating a salad, and instead go for a pizza, or something in that category.

It also gives you time for contemplating and for adopting personal change. You will learn more about this in the next topic that will be discussed dafter thing, however, when you are running you tend to strengthen your resolve to become healthy. Also, when you work so hard every single day to keep your calories and fat off, then you also do not overeat so that all your hard work does not go to waste in any way. There are several benefits to jogging and to running so you can really pick the one of your choice and start incorporating this habit in your life.

3. Cycling

You may think that cycling only takes care of the lower half of the body just as you thought that pushups only take care of the upper half of the body but 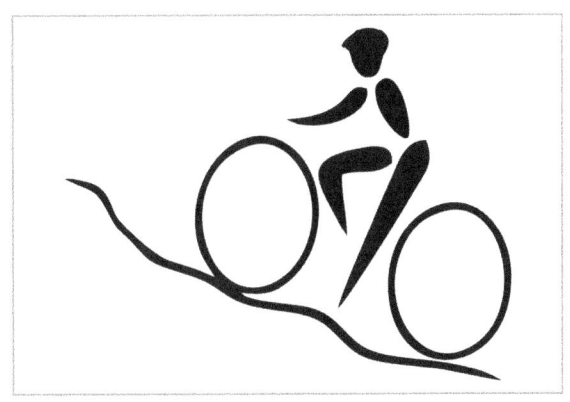 just as it was untrue for the pushups; it is untrue for cycling as well. When you cycle, the biggest favor you are doing yourself is getting rid of body fat concentrated in your thighs, your legs and your belly. This means that when you cycle you can hope for a flat belly and for you to lose weight easily.

When you cycle you can do it at home at a stationary cycle but you can also purchase one in real and cycle your way to work. This means that you save time and you do not have to actually take out some time for the gym if you do either of these things. When you cycle to work, you can save time and still get a lot of exercise done without sweating and without having to dedicate time to take a shower before you get to work. If you are riding a stationary cycle you can do so while reading a book, watching a movie or doing anything at all. When you ride a cycle you can accomplish so much at the same time.

When you cycle the core of your body is automatically addressed and made use of. When you core comes into play losing weight becomes easier because it makes sure your entire body is involved in the action. When the center of gravity of your body gives you the strength to carry on with the exercise, the muscles all over your body derive the strength from the core and then get involved in the action. This allows you to lose weight and become toned and fit.

4. Lunges

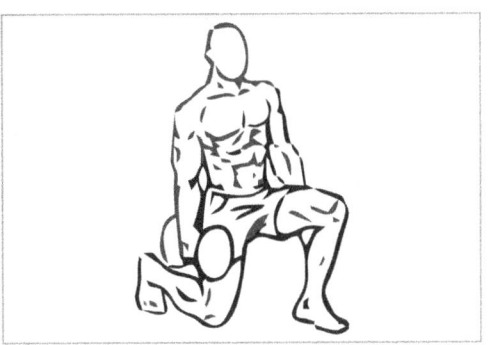

Lunges are difficult to do, we get it. They are also painful and sometimes you have to muster a little more energy for them that we think helps us at all. However, doing lunges is more effective than half of the other exercises combined. The speed with which you lose weight when you are doing lunges is actually remarkable because when you move your legs, and place your weight on different legs according to the movements, you are using your core again.

This enables your muscles to become stronger, to burn fat and the calories that have been stored in the same muscles. By doing lunges you can address the stored fat and calories in the thighs, the legs and even the calf area. Moreover, you can also make your belly look flat in no time by doing lunges frequently.

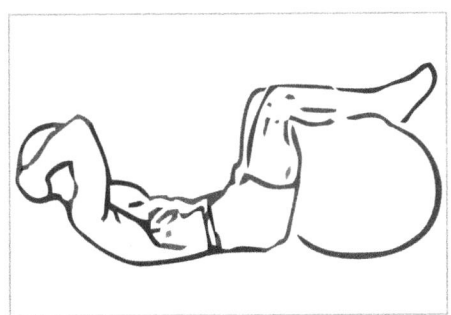

5. Crunches

Crunches are effective and they make your arms and your shoulders look amazing. They take some effort but they get the job done when it comes to it. When you do crunches, you are once again addressing your core. We cannot emphasize on how important it is to engage the core of your body and to play it out in the rest of your muscles. You will never really have the strength to carry out even the simplest of exercises for long if you do not locate and use your core to accomplish them.

6. Mountain Climbers

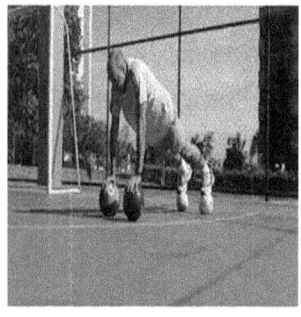 These are very effective when it comes to toning the muscles of your body. If you find them to be a little too hard for you then you can easily do what you did with the pushups; start small and then finish big. You can also try to move your legs slowly at first and then move on to the advanced level in a gradual manner. Mountain climbers make your belly flat, your back toned and your legs supple. Your arms also derive some strength, they also become supple and your shoulders also let go of the fat and calories stored in there. This type of exercise is very good for your entire body.

You can do mountain climbers in your home on a yoga mat as well. You do not have to go to the gym and do that at a class alone. You can do them at home, play on some fast music to motivate you and then get on with it. Keep on thinking that

www.puredietweightloss.com

you can do it, and unless you complete it do not let yourself stop. However, keep yourself away from injury and do not push yourself unnecessarily far. As we have already mentioned before, take it slow and opt for baby steps instead of giant and unrealistic leaps that will not become a permanent part of your lifestyle.

Do I Need A Special Trainer?

In one word- no. You do not need a special trainer in order to be fit and thin. In fact, it would be a lot better for you to be your own special trainer and see what you do to regulate your diet and your exercise regimen on your own. Since most people are of the opinion that they will not be able to continue with the routine unless they find a trainer to motivate them, they believe it is important to get a trainer and to have a strict schedule. However, you have to be your own special trainer because no one can watch you like you do and no one really knows your body as best as you do.

This means that having a trainer is not going to help you if you just decide to help yourself. Will power is an ingrained thing in the human psyche and it is part of everybody's character and personality. You just have to know how to truly tap into your potential and gain access to that large reservoir of will power and sheer grit and determination.

It is not rally that hard to follow through when it comes to that, Many people find it easier to follow through once they know they rely on themselves and that they are their own kind of trainer who programs their diet and their exercise regimen according to what they body actually needs instead of just following a generic principal that may or may not apply to them.

This goes for women and men when they want to lose weight because it may seem like having a special trainer makes things easier but it really does not. When another person starts having an influence in your personal life and on things such as what you eat, what you drink and what you do with your free time then you start becoming more and unhappy with your life. You lose that sense of freedom you love so much. When you are told what you have to do instead of deciding yourself like a mature adult, you start depending on the trainer and when they are out of sight there is a very high probability that you may end up cheating on your diet plan.

People with a lower level of will power can develop it without having to depend on someone else to get the job done. They can start off small and then build on from that, such as starting off from the will power of not eating chocolate or reducing the amount of sugar drunk in coffee or in tea. These people will build will power as you built stamina in the exercises that have been stated and explained above. Stamina and will power are things that can be increased if you really want to do it.

You do not really need a trainer for yourself; you just need confidence and very high self-esteem so that when you are alone with yourself and your thoughts you know that you will not cheat on your diet just because you yourself said it so. In that way, your trainer will always be you and will never leave your side. This is also a trainer that will constantly nag you when you feel like skipping exercise or eating something very unhealthy. If you are your own special trainer then you can accomplish something that no one else can, you can incorporate healthy food not your lifestyle and establish a proper exercise regimen so that no matter what you do or where you go you can continue with that on your own without any kind of external help.

When Exercise and Diet Doesn't Work

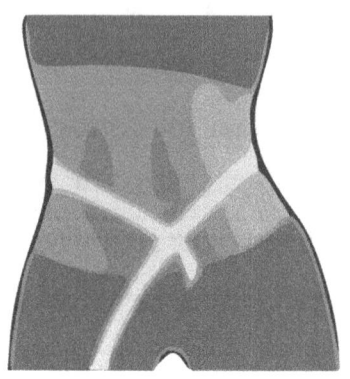

Many people wonder why exactly exercise and diet do not work as they expect them to work. When you start eating healthy for a change, you start assuming that the weight you have gained over all this time will start dropping off rather soon. Even if it does drop initially you will note that it will stay stuck at one point or another and it will refuse to be off your body unless you do something more. This is due to one reason that no one else has considered as yet; the psychology of weight loss.

The Psychology of Weight Loss

The psychology of weight loss is something that encompasses two important factors of losing weight, one of which is a strict exercise and diet regimen whereas the other refers to something that people do not consider important for weight loss; personal change. Unless you incorporate personal change in your personality and in your outlook towards life you will never be able to lose the weight you want to lose at this moment.

To accomplish anything in life you have to incorporate change in the foundation of your thinking and your personality. You have to have perseverance and adherence to the rules to see your mission through till the very end. If you change your pattern of thinking you are bound to accomplish so much more than you have ever done before in your life.

Self-Control

Self-control is an important part of everyone's personality that is not only applied in the weight loss aspect of life, but in all spheres of our day to day lives. This includes the self-control you apply in your life when you wish to procrastinate but have to study, or when you control your temper or control the urge to smoke or drink. You can accomplish this tough goal by focusing on what will happen if you do not stop from doing it. Instead of focusing on what amount of weight you will gain when you start eating imagine how much weight you are bound to lose if you skip this one thing you are a little tempted to eat. This can help you achieve self-control like you have never been able to do before.

Positive Thinking

The power of positive thinking is so profound and so paramount that scientists, psychologists and spiritual scholars are still unable to define it in a demographic. Nevertheless, positive thinking is something that can improve not only your outlook on the situation but also the result of the particular situation. Your positive thoughts are like vibes that you send out into the universe, and many research studies have clearly and most definitely shown that the vibes you send out into the universe come back to you reflected in the same capacity as you sent them out in the first place. This means that if you do send out positive thoughts, then good things are bound to happen to you however, if you absolve and give up in the face of negativity then you will obviously be receiving that negativity reflected back at you.

Family Support

This factor is not that much recognized but it comes into play a lot of the time because whenever you do something or set yourself on the journey to 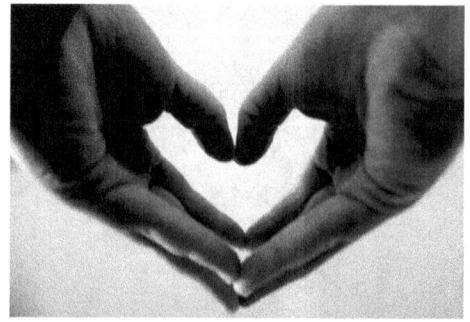 accomplish something you look back at your family members your friends and your teachers to give you some sense of appreciation or encouragement. As human beings we are conditioned to accept the love and the praise of the people who are closets to us and the people who we tend to trust. This means that when you are trying to watch your weight, if your family becomes an immense source of respect for you, you will have a better time of handling the bad times and coping with them than you would have had if your family had been unsupportive of your ways.

There is also the very well understood fact that people who do not tell their families they are on such a regimen and are working and planning to lose a bunch of weight, tend to be faced with delicious irresistible and tempting meals when they visit family. In that moment of euphoria it could easily be forgotten what your mission is. Your will power could dissolve and there would be no one near you to help you regain that will power.

When you family is aware of your predicament they make extra efforts to make sure this process is as easy for you as they can make it out to be. They are here to facilitate you in your quest to attain fitness and health and they do not want any obstacles in your way. This would mean that family and friends who support people in their family trying to lose weight, tend to be closer to that particular person than families who do not support the idea in the first place.

There is another class of relations that deal with this situation in a very bad way. Sometimes people try to taunt the other person to lose weight instead of talking to them nicely about it. Sometimes they try to put them down just because of their weight or because their body shape is different from what is supposed to be normal. This may not be a practice followed by your initial family members but some other relatives tend to have these habits too. It is always best to stay away from these people even in the best of circumstances let alone circumstances such as these. Your family is your rock and your support system and it is best to seek their support in a time such as this.

How Do I Lose Weight with the Right Kind of Attitude?

When you lose weight, as mentioned above, you have to have the right kind of attitude to do it. What you think and how you phrase your thoughts is essential to the cause. This means that even if you think "I cannot do it" add a "yet" to the end of the sentence. The stronger you are in your thoughts the stronger you are going to be in your resolve. You have to think thoughts such as "I am in the right place to lose some weight this year",

"I am hopping and ready to get into shape", "I have to stop making excuses and start looking the way I want to look". There is also the sense of purpose that comes with these thoughts.

When you want to get thinner only because you want to look better, you will realize you will get thinner faster. If you are doing it to make other people happy you will understand that you will never be able to lose weight. You will also be miserable and very much tempted to cheat on your diet and exercise routine. Whenever you do something in life that ends up making you happy and satisfied with your actions you are more likely to succeed. This is why losing weight is a psychological game more than a physical one. Here are a few things that you have to consider when you are trying to lose some weight:

You have to find what motivates you

Whenever you get down to doing something you have to figure out what motivates you or inspires you. Make a list of things and conduct small experiments to see what drives you to accomplish your goals. Try to sit alone and think about all your previous accomplishments and how you came to achieving them. What have you previously done in the face of adversity that has helped you achieve the impossible or the difficult? Here are a few things to consider if you are still having some trouble coming up with something that motivates you.

- When someone tells you that you cannot do something does that motivate you to prove them wrong?

- When you see someone with a good toned body do you think I am going to look like that as well?

- Realizing that without pain and hard work you would not gain anything

- Work hard for a week and have a cheat day at the end of the week to reward yourself

- Set up your exercise routine and tell yourself if you finish it you can watch an episode of your favorite TV show

- Listen to songs while exercising so that you lose track of time and do not count down every single second which makes the time seem longer and unbearable

- You can also work out while watching TV or reading a book so that you do not count down every single second which makes the time seem longer and unbearable

What Affects Your Weight Loss Psychology

Like all things in life, your mind frame affects your actions on a great level. There are many numerous factors that affect your actions and these all 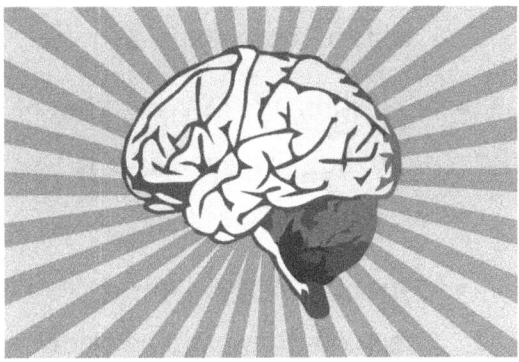 come from your mind and your psyche. Here are a few questions that you have to ask yourself to ensure that you are not being held back by your thoughts and that you can bring yourself to accomplish anything that you really want to accomplish:

- Question No. 1: What motivates you to do something that you know is going to be difficult?

- Question No. 2: What are the factors that cause you to fail instead of succeeding?

- Question No. 3: How do you learn from these failures and what to do you to make sure that you do not fail in the same way again?

- Question No. 4: How do I set realistic goals?

- Question No. 5: How do I make sure that I implement these practices and goals in my life and how do I achieve those goals?

- Question No. 6: What kind of a personality do you have and how can you use it to your advantage for losing weight fast?

- Question No. 7: How do you maintain this attitude and keep off the weight as well?

- Question No. 8: What is your opinion about yourself?

- Question No. 9: What are your habits and your patterns of behavior and how do you avoid falling into the same traps over and over again when it comes to losing weight?

- Question No. 10: Do you have any personal conflicts that you are facing at the moment?

When you ask and answer these questions yourself you will reach a new level of self-awareness. Just as you sat down and figured out what motivates you, you have to sit down and answer all of these other questions as well. Try to be as honest with yourself as it is possible because being honest is going to help you immensely in this case.

The more you motivate yourself to do something the stronger you get and the more your resolve strengthens. With proper exercise and eating a proper diet and the right kind of attitude you can achieve your standard goal of weight loss without crash dieting.

When you start losing weight, you will find it easier to follow the diet and exercise regimen however, as the days pass by you will find it harder to do so. This is why maintaining a strong resolve, keeping up happy thoughts and being determined will help you along the way of seeing it through right until the very end. This kind of attitude will also help you keep the weight off and maintain the weight you have reached after working so hard for so long. This is why the psychology of losing weight plays an immense role in taking off the weight and keeping it off as well.

Lose Fat, Gain Muscles

You can easily starve yourself and lose weight without eating anything at all but that is not recommended because it could either develop into an eating disorder or it could have adverse effects on your body. Your health is of utmost importance which is why being in shape comes secondary to having good and sound health. Your immune system, your digestive system and your muscles are the most affected when you cut food from your life and go on a crash diet. It is only smart to consider the alternative of eating healthy and keeping up with the nutritional balance that your body needs to function.

There are many ways of making sure that you lose weight and most of them are unhealthy. This does not mean that any of them are easy; it only means that they give you quicker results and end up causing harm to your body instead. You should worry about your strength and you muscles and develop them despite burning the fat that is stored in your body. Here are a few tips you can follow to make sure that when you do lose weight, you do not lose your muscles alongside it.

- Tip # 1: Eat Enough Portions of Protein

We all know proteins build muscles and these are present in meat even though there are some vegetarian options such as beans. Never give up proteins completely, although it's best to eat them in moderation. Do not eat harmful kinds of meat and instead go for poultry, mince meat and fish.

- Tip # 2: Eat Proper Food Before a Workout

When you think of working out do not starve yourself before it. Give yourself enough energy by consuming proper, healthy and energetic food so that you can develop your muscles instead of exerting them.

- Tip # 3: Eat Proper Food After a Workout

After a workout do not just give up on food completely. When you work hard in a workout it's completely natural to give up eating after the workout but have a proper meal an hour or so after you have gone through with it. This gives your body the nutrition it needs in order to build and develop your muscles and to make them stronger than they were before.

- Tip # 4: Don't completely give up on calories

Many people think giving up on calories is the ultimate solution; well, it's not! Watch your calories because each and every one of us is required to take in some amount of calories every day. Make sure these are good calories and not calories that contain fat. These will make you stronger without making you fatter.

- Tip # 5: Take Diet Breaks as Well

Most popularly recognized as a cheat day concept, take some diet breaks so that your body can have a different atmosphere as well. It needs some variety and some change and one special meal in two weeks is not going to be the end of the world. Just know when to stop and what to stop at and you will be fine.

- Tip # 6: Do not Overdose on Cardio

Cardio is great for losing weight, but the catch is that cardio effectively burns fat and calories without doing too much for the muscles in your body. It only makes them lean and does not make them strong. You can mix and match exercises such as conducting 5 minutes of strength exercises (pushups, mountain climbers and presses), with 3 minutes of Cardio and something like that. Combining exercises is always very effective for building muscles and losing weight.

- Tip # 7: Eat Only Healthy and Clean Food

Do not eat junk food or friend food or food that can have a bad effect on your body. Eat clean food and healthy food that will go in and make your body feel good from the inside. Your body is like a machine and it will not function properly if the substances you insert in it are not good for it. Instead, the body systems will start slowing down and there will be several cogs in the machine if you do not take proper care of it.

- Tip # 8: Conserve Your Carbohydrates

Do not try to immediately burn your carbs if you consume them, conserve them because they are a valid source of energy. If you have to fear anything, fear fats don't fear carbs. If taken in the right amount they can do wonders for your health. Giving up completely on carbohydrates is never a good idea so try not to be a little extreme when you diet and opt for moderation instead.

- Tip # 9: Although Never Eat Carbs Without a Complementary Dish

Never have carbohydrates on an empty stomach always pair them up with some sort of vegetable, protein or something like that. It makes sure that the carbohydrates are used for energy instead of being stored in the form of fat by the body. Pair up bread with a few cabbages, a light soup or something delicious so that you can have your daily dose of carbohydrates but by complementing them with another nutrient component that will distract your body from the carbs you are taking in. Your body should have carbohydrates for the use of energy and when they go in, you should make sure that they are used up as energy and not stored as fats.

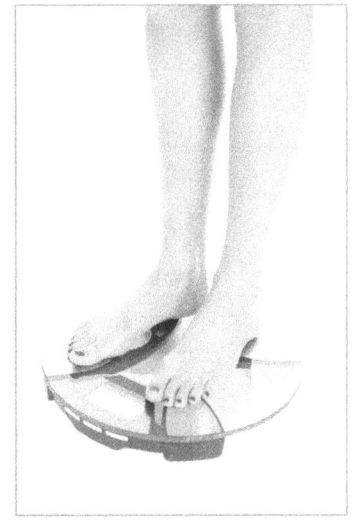

- Tip # 10: Do Not Consume Carbs Before Bed

When you sleep your metabolic system goes down a substantial amount which is why the body stops consuming energy and starts storing it instead. This is the main reason as to why people insist that you should not have large meals before you go to sleep. This is also the reason why you should not eat fats or carbohydrates when you go to sleep, since your body will store them up in the form of fats and your muscle strength will not go up at all.

ACTION STEPS

1. Get access to my 10-part Paleo Diet Mini Course at www.puredietweightloss.com

2. Prepare your new recipes.

3. Start eating and living a healthier life.

How to Retain Your Loss

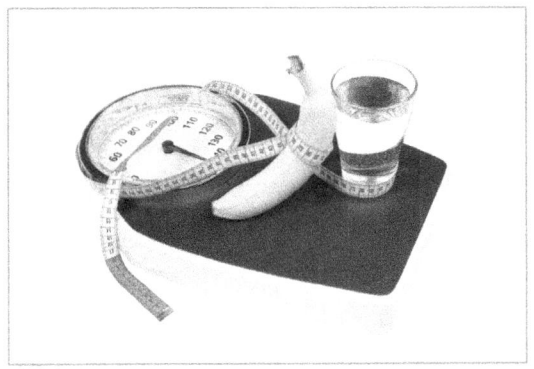 Were you able to shed the extra 112 pounds successfully through your weight loss plan and diet? If so, do not think that your struggle ends here. For those who were not able to lose the desired weight with the diet or exercise plan, worry not. If your diet and exercise plan is flawless, then you might not have the motivation to pursue your weight loss goals. This section will help you discover the ways to reduce your weight through motivation.

The power of Motivation

Motivation is one of the powerful elements that can make people accomplish impossible tasks. It's motivation that allows your brain to act according to your in-depth desires. It is motivation that prepares your brain to endure the pain of exercise programs. If you understand how to use motivation, you can easily retain your weight loss and maintain your perfect slim figure.

So what exactly is motivation?

"Motivation is the reason behind our actions."

Why do you get out of bed in the early morning? What makes you dress up and go to work? Motivation is the reason behind all our actions. In one way or the other motivation is always involved with our daily life. The challenge is to use your motivational force to achieve your weight loss goals. Sometimes people feel that they cannot get themselves to the gym just because they do not feel like it.

Many people face this problem where they do not feel motivated enough to exercise. Why do you go to work every day? Because you know that you have to earn a decent living to pay your bills and maintain a lifestyle so you can survive in the society. Similarly, you have to persuade yourself that you need to lose your weight to maintain a healthy lifestyle.

How does it Work?

This is the most important question: how do you achieve the right motivation? There are

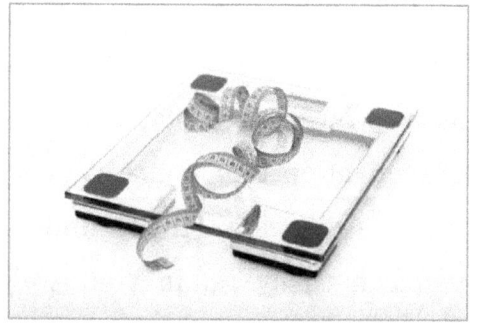

several ways that can help you achieve the right motivation to work out. Many people quit gym after they have reached the desired weight, which is a wrong practice. First of all keep in mind that:

- Losing 112 pounds quickly does not mean you cannot gain them back

- Ignoring your diet and exercise after weight loss can make you gain weight faster

- Without weight maintenance your body can become prone to various diseases

It is very important that you understand the risks involved in gaining weight after the weight loss. You have to keep going for the rest of your life so you can never have that obesity nightmare again. Here is a list of things that can keep you motivated through your life to maintain a healthy weight:

- Write a mission statement: Write down your weight loss goals with a reason; why you need to achieve a certain goal. Read this mission statement every day. Place it somewhere where you can easily read it. For example, you can paste the mission statement on your fridge or bedroom door, so you can have maximum exposure to it.

Your mission statement can be something like: I need to lose 60 pounds so I can fit in my mother's wedding dress.

If you have achieved your desired figure, your mission statement could be: *I want to look like   this after ten years.*

- Make smaller goals: If you need to lose a lot of weight, start with small goals. You cannot shed 6-10 pounds in a week, so make smaller, weekly goals that would help you reduce 2-5 pounds a week at least.

- Control your urge to eat: After you have a mission statement and a plan, make sure that you curb your urge to eat more than you need. Most people use candy and other sugary foods as snacks, which is an extremely dangerous practice that can lead to large accumulation of fat.

- Take your Picture: This is the best motivational trick ever. Take your picture in a b   ikini. Do you like the way your body looks? If 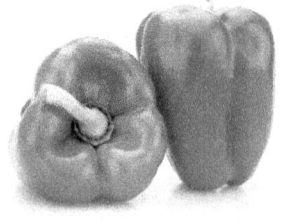 not, then let this picture be the reminder and a motivation. Take a picture in a way that it shows off your body completely. You should be able to learn about the areas that have excessive cellulite, so you can work on them individually. Most commonly, thighs become the victim of cellulite.

In case you have achieved your desired weight, then take a picture to remind yourself that you want to look like this for the rest of your life.

- Monitor your progress: Your mission and picture would provide you ample motivation to go on with your diet and exercise program. Monitor your progress and compare yourself to your last picture to make sure that you are on track.

I am Motivated but I still don't feel like I should stick to the plan

If you do not feel like that you should stick to the plan even when you feel that you are motivated, then there two possible things that can be wrong:

1. Your plan might not be flexible or achievable enough for you to follow

2. You might not be motivated enough

So, look into both the things and figure out what's wrong. If your plan is not attainable, then break down your goals into mini achievable goals that are easy to follow on a regular basis. Some people try to force their bodies to go through vigorous and hard core exercises that are hard to complete on a regular basis. This drastically impacts your motivation and even though you want to keep going, your body does not allow you to go through with it.

Find a plan that is easy to follow. The goal should not be to exhaust the body, but rather it should focus on developing physical strength while trimming the fat.

Understand your Hunger cue

So now that you are motivated enough to reach certain weight loss goals and you have the plan to work through, let's understand how you can curb your hunger.

Can you distinguish between the real hunger and just the need to eat? Many people who suffer from obesity find it hard to identify their hunger cue. Research shows that people who take more snacks and larger meals a day eventually develop a habit of eating more than they need. Before we dig further into this topic, let's first understand why people need to eat more and what psychological factors are involved behind this act.

Why we eat more than we need?

Most scientific studies suggest that the impulse to eat more arises from our brain, not stomach. Scientific research shows that people who have low quantity of receptors in their brain cells for dopamine, a hormone that is responsible to induce the feelings of satisfaction and wellness. Most eating disorders are related to the lack of dopamine.

People who suffer a lack of dopamine find it hard to resist temptations and usually overeat. Overeating is usually a pleasurable experience for people and can be hard to treat. In addition, people who overeat hardly understand the consequences of overeating. Before we go any further, let's understand the concepts of needs, wants and desires and how they contribute towards abnormal eating patterns.

Need: Need is characterized by an individual's functional necessity that includes a proper, nutritional meal for the well-being of the body. Need can easily transform into a want and desire if the person suffers of overeating disorder or simply fails to curb his hunger.

As mentioned above, hunger can easily be stretched; you can get your body used to consuming 7-8 slices of pizza at a time if you make it a habit. At first, your body might resist the change, but over time it will surrender to the level of consumption. The challenge is to keep your needs controlled by resisting the temptations to eat more.

Want: Want refers to the body's need to consume something that is desirable. If you usually eat a red velvet cupcake after a proper meal, it is very likely that you are consuming it because you want it, not because you need. When you hear people say "I want a cup of coffee," it means that they would like to have a cup of coffee, but they don't necessarily need it. Once you learn to distinguish the thin line between wanting something and needing something, you can easily control your appetite.

As mentioned above, the excess need to eat arises from your mind, not your stomach. So, in order to control your hunger, it is important that you learn about your hunger cue; when so you really get hungry? In addition, it is also important to recognize when your stomach is full. Research suggests that people who eat less than they need usually enjoy better health than people who keep their stomachs full.

Desire: Desire is an outcome of want. Most people become the victim of obesity just because of their uncontrollable desires to overeat. Desires can lead to substantial weight gain, which is why it's important to learn about your hunger cue.

How do I control my hunger?

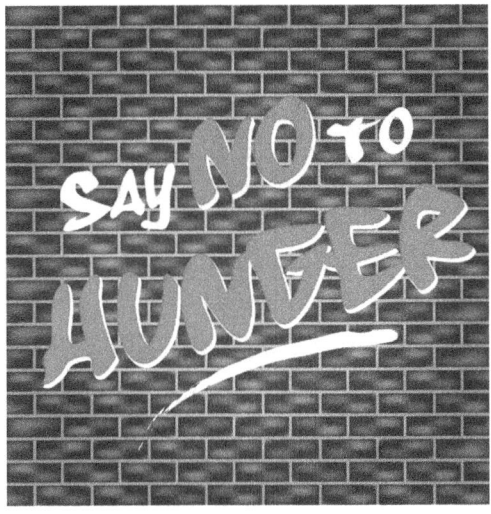

Hunger and sleep are the two characteristics of the body that can be controlled. All you have to do is set your body's clock and follow the pattern without any disruptions. There are three most important factors that contribute towards hunger control, namely, motivation, control and determination. First of all, understand that if you will not curb your hunger today, you will have to a bigger price few years later. Gaining weight is far easier than losing weight, so curb your hunger today to avoid weight problems in the future.

Below is the well-sorted list of things that can help you curb your hunger:

- The leafy green salad: There is no denying that fruits and vegetables are the best option to consume a healthy diet without any worry about the weight again. Instead of having a processed snack in a coffee break, try a leafy green salad and curb your hunger. Research shows that green vegetables keep you full for longer in contrast to the processed snacks.

- Reduce appetite with grapefruit: According to various research studies, grapefruit is rich in fiber, which helps your body feel less hungry than it usually does. In addition, other foods such as orange, bran, peas and whole grains also help you curb your appetite.

- Try low fat dairy foods: Research suggests that low fat dairy products are a great way to get the nutritional strength without attaining the additional fat that accumulates in the body over time causing obesity.

So there you have it, the most effective ways that can help your curb your hunger. Keep in mind that curbing your hunger has nothing to do with dieting. Most people starve themselves in order to avoid gaining extra pounds. The key is to eat healthy and avoid overeating

Once you learn the difference between getting hunger and feeling hunger, you will be able to control your hunger.

Feeling hungry vs. getting hungry

"Feeling hungry" is not exactly a genuine hunger. As mentioned above, feeling hungry is a psychological factor that motivates us to consume additional food. 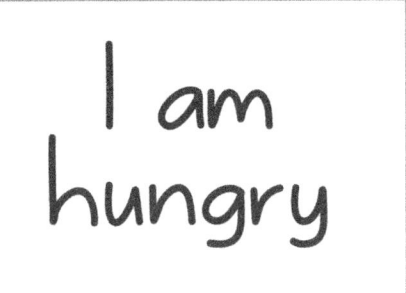 The motivation for eating more can arise from various factors. Most commonly, people feel hungry when they are bored and feel that eating might help you keep your mind busy. Scientific studies suggest that most Americans are overeating due to the heavy advertising and promotion of commercial products that are hard to resist.

To make sure that you don't fall for the "feeling hungry" trap, schedule your diet. For example, you can have three full meals and two snacks a day with high fiber and low fat dairy food. It is recommended not to have more than a single course of desert throughout the day. Only have more than one course of dessert if it is low in fat and sugar.

The Ultimate Reward

If you have been committed to your diet and exercise program for a while, you will notice the improved body contours along with numerous health benefits. Apart from a healthy, slim physique, maintaining your weight offers countless benefits. Some of these benefits include:

- Reduced risk of heart disease: American heart association report showed a survey result that proves that weight maintenance keep the heart healthy and reduces the risks of various heart related diseases.

- Reduced risk of cancer: Research shows that weight maintenance reduces the risk of various forms of cancer, including skin cancer and lung cancer.

- Reduced risk of diabetes: The major cause of type II diabetes is obesity. Weight maintenance helps you reduce the risk of type II diabetes.

- Reduced risk of rheumatic diseases: Obesity is one of the major causes of rheumatic diseases that are, most of the time, incurable. A healthy weight ensures that your body does not become a victim of rheumatic diseases such as arthritis and osteoarthritis.

- Reduced risk of infertility: Research shows that weight maintenance reduces the risks of infertility in women. The balanced diet and the proper exercise, keep the organs healthy that allow easy fertilization.

- More self-confidence and self-esteem: When you look healthy and feel healthy, you automatically feel more confident. One of the major benefits of weight maintenance is its ability to equip you with a sound confidence and self-esteem that can help you do better in life.

- Increased physical energy: Diet and exercise, build muscular strength which contributes towards the overall physical strength. Healthy body contains a healthy mind, which helps you lead a better life.

According to a research study, the right exercise and diet helped countless people reduce their dress sizes. In addition, according to the American heart association, people who exercise are less prone to heart related diseases than others.

I don't feel like I have been rewarded

If you feel like that even after a year of workout you have seen no substantial results, it is quite possible that your diet or exercise plan don't resonate well with your body's parameters. Have you tried changing your diet or exercise plan? Most people make the mistake of getting on with the plan without any expert consultation. If you suffer from any disorders, you must first consult your health specialist.

Work with your specialist to find a diet and exercise plan that would work best for your body. Not every diet works for everybody, so find what suits you the best and start over again. Remember do not let anything demotivate you. Use the motivation tips discussed above to find your motivation to achieve your weight loss goal.

Sometimes you may fail to notice a difference if the change is minor. Even if your body fails to shed weight, exercise and diet will still be helping you from the inside. You might notice the difference at first, but slowly you will start to witness the transformation. So keep going and wait for the day when you will finally get your dream figure.

Apple Cider Vinegar for Weight Loss

Acids are very helpful in the digestion of protein, which enables you to lose weight all the while being aided by the digestion process. If you increase your intake of apple cider vinegar, you can digest the proteins at work in the body for producing some vital hormones; since proteins are basically involved in the production of hormones.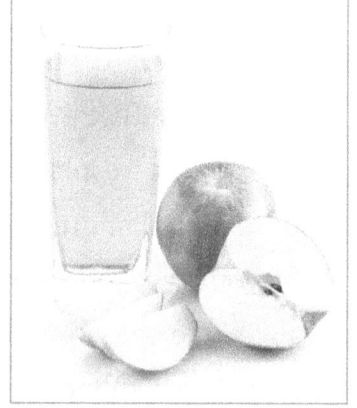

This means that the hormones that play an active part in increasing metabolic activity in your body tend to increase in number, and hence your metabolic rate also increases. Due to the fact that it helps break down proteins and helps with the digestion process, it also allows fats to stay in the body for a far less time.

The fats that is stored in the body, when encounter the elements of apple cider vinegar, break down and stay in the body for a lesser amount of time than they would have otherwise. This means that the body will lose fats at a faster rate and it will also make you healthy since apple cider vinegar cuts through fats and gives you the opportunity to have the kind of body that you want.

There is another element that is digested quickly when you drink apple cider vinegar and that element is iron. When you have more iron in your body the oxygen cells will be transferred around your body at a faster rate which means that you will lose weight faster. Oxygen is an essential element which plays a vital part in burning the energy components in your body. This means that the carbohydrates you consume will not be stored in the body instead they will be utilized for energy and will make you healthy.

Green Tea for Weight Loss

You might have heard millions of times that green tea is an

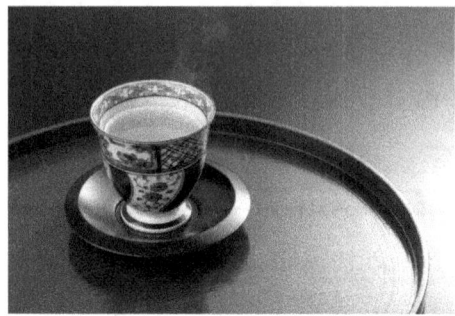

essential ingredient in weight loss. When you are thinking of losing weight you can add green tea to your daily schedule and it does wonders to keep you in shape. For some people it proves to be a little more effective which enables them to eat whatever they want as long as they consume green tea on a daily basis. For others, it works at a slower rate which means that they also have to watch their diet while incorporating a cup or two of green tea in their day to day lives.

Green tea is a detoxifier which means that when you consume it your body will not only lose weight but it is also bound to become cleaner and healthier. Your muscles will lose the extra and unwanted material that is stored in them (also inclusive of fat) and your vital organs will also start functioning properly. This is one of

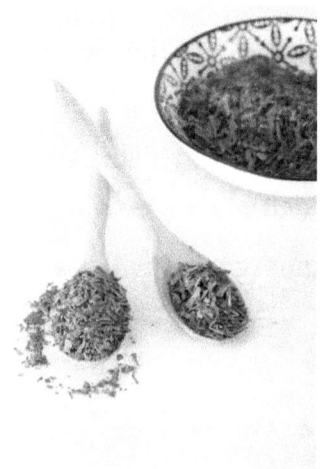

the reasons as to why your digestion increases and it also boosts your metabolic activity.

When you consume green tea, you have to be aware of the fact that it cuts through the fat in your muscles. This means that the fat you try so hard to get rid of can be dissolved by consuming green tea on a daily basis. By consuming green tea you can also reduce your chances of eating junk food and snacks which are the primary reason as to why you have gained so much weight. It gets rid of the hunger pangs and effectively fills your stomach with nutrients and elements that prove to be good for your body. This type of drink is also often referred to as a drink with negative calories as you can minus the calories and benefit from other advantages it presents at the same time.

Recipes for Better Shape and Health

When it comes to weight loss, finding the right combination of fruits and vegetable can be hard. This section covers some tantalizing natural juice recipes that can help you gain the nutrition that your body needs while you lose the extra pounds.

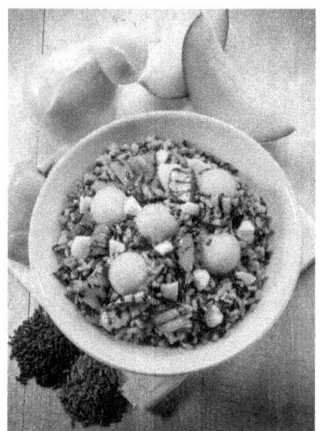

Enticing recipes for losing weight without losing body strength

Here are the most effective juice recipes that have been proven to provide excellent results for people who are trying to shed a few pounds.

Orange and Parsley Juice

Ingredients for the Orange and Parsley juice

- Oranges (5-6 for one glass of juice)

- 1 cup of parsley (you can increase or decrease the amount)

Preparing the juice:

1. Peel the oranges and remove their seeds. Make sure that the oranges you picked are fresh and ripe.

2. Thoroughly rinse parsley in the water and place it in the blender/juicer with the oranges after it is dried.

3. Pour the contents of the juicer into a glass and consume.

How does it help me reduce weight?

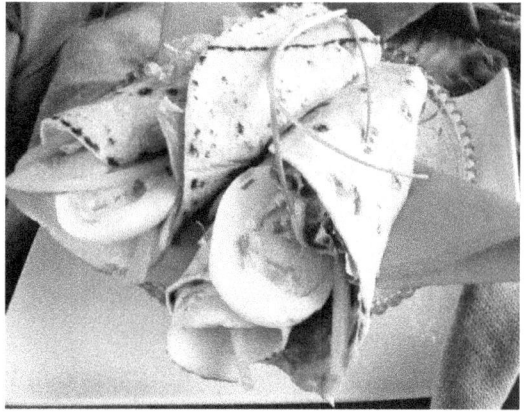

Both the ingredients offer a low calorie diet that keeps your stomach full for longer. You feel full and satisfied and can easily resist the temptation to overeat. Orange is rich in vitamin C, which helps you reduce your appetite and ultimately reduce your weight. Parsley, on the other hand, is a fiber rich natural ingredient that can be a perfect replacement for processed snacks. Parsley usually consumed with other fruits and vegetables. Parsley is full of Vitamins (A, C and K) that are essential for overall physical endurance.

Apple, Carrot and Celery Juice

Ingredients for the Apple, Carrot and Celery Juice

- Two apples

- Two carrots

- 4 -5 stalks of celery

Preparing the juice:

1. Thoroughly rinse the apples, carrots and celery.

2. You can peel the apples if you wish, but usually it is not necessary. Apple peel contains vitamins and antioxidants that are healthy for health; therefore, it is advisable to leave them as it is. Cut the apples into smaller pieces.

3. Peel the carrots and chop them into smaller pieces.

4. Chop the celery stalks into small sticks.

5. Place the ingredients into the juicer and blend.

6. Pour the juice into your glass and enjoy a healthy, nutritious drink.

How does it help me reduce weight?

The goodness of natural fruit and vegetables gives you more physical endurance while you work out to reduce your weight.

Pear, Ginger and Celery Juice

Another great nutritious drink is created with a combination of Pear, Ginger and Celery.

Ingredients for the Pear, Ginger and Celery Juice
- Chopped pear slices (1 bowl)

- A large celery stalk

- A ginger root

Preparing the juice:
1. Wash the ingredients under the tap water.

2. Peel of the ginger root (do not use more than 1-inch of the root)

3. Chop the celery stalk into smaller pieces.

4. Now, place the ingredients in the juicer and blend.

5. Pour the juice into your favorite glass and enjoy.

How does it help me reduce weight?

Research shows that pears are great natural laxatives that allow easy digestion. Celery and ginger also help with digestion and allow you to have a balanced stomach.

Banana, Melon and Apple Juice

Ingredients for the Banana, Melon and Apple Juice

- 2-3 bananas

- One raw melon (bitter)

- 2-4 apples

- ½ Glass of distilled water

Preparing the juice:

1. Wash the ingredients thoroughly.

2. Peel the bananas and chop them into small pieces.

3. Peel the melon and slice it into smaller pieces.

4. Chop the apple into smaller parts.

5. Blend the ingredients in a juicer along with distilled water and enjoy the natural goodness of fruits.

How does it help me reduce weight?

Melon is a great ingredient for body detoxification. In addition, research has shown that melon can reduce the fat accumulation in the body over time and help you gain the figure of your dreams. Bananas are rich in potassium and vitamins that give the body its needed strength.

Mango, Banana, Spinach and Peach Juice

Ingredients for the Mango, Banana, Spinach and Peach Juice

- 1-2 mangoes

- A ripe banana

- Spinach (1 bowl)

- 1-2 peaches

- Distilled water

Preparing the juice:

1. Peel the mango skin and separate the juicy part from the seed.

2. Peel the bananas and chop them into smaller pieces.

3. Cut the peaches in smaller slices.

4. Place all the ingredients in the juicer along with the distilled water.

5. Pour the drink and have nourishing refreshment.

How does it help me reduce weight?

All the ingredients in this recipe are rich in potassium, fiber, antioxidants and amino acids that not only help you improve your overall health, but also allow you to reduce weight. This juice can be great if taken after exercise.

Orange, Beet, Mint and Carrot Juice

Ingredients for the Orange, Beet, Mint and Carrot Juice

- 1-2 oranges

- 2-3 carrots (medium size)

- 1 beetroot

- Mint leaves (around 8)

Preparing the juice:

1. Just like always, wash the ingredients before the process.

2. Peel off the oranges and the carrots and chop them down into smaller slices.

3. Chop of the roots and the green part of the beet root and cut into smaller pieces.

4. Place the mint, carrots, beet root and orange into the juicer and blend.

5. Enjoy an energizing drink for a better health.

How does it help me reduce weight?

The beetroot and mint offer powerful nutrients and antioxidants that keep your strength up while you exercise. The nutrients of this juice help you maintain a healthy weight even after you have achieved your desired weight. Scientific research shows that beetroot is a great ingredient for weight loss. Include beetroot in your diet and get the figure of your dreams faster. In addition, the beetroot also helps you flush out the toxins in the body that can lead to less than favorable physical health.

Pineapple, Carrot, Chili and Lime Juice

Ingredients for the Pineapple, Carrot, Chili and Lime Juice

- 1 pineapple chopped in chunks

- 1-2 carrots, chopped or sliced

- ½ Teaspoon of lime juice

- 1-2 green or red chili

- 2-3 ice cubes

Preparing the juice:

1. Wash all the ingredients thoroughly with cold water.

2. Peel off the extra skin of the carrots and pineapple and chop them down into small slices.

3. Place the ingredients in the juicer and add the lime juice and the ice cubes.

4. Blend properly and consume.

How does it help me reduce weight?

This recipe provides a juice packed with vitamins and nutrients that are necessary for the growth of body and mind. Pineapple and chili are a great source of antioxidants that enhance your metabolism and ultimately improve your digestion. Strong metabolism never allows your body to accumulate extra fat, which gives you a perfect figure that you desire.

Kiwi, Pineapple, Broccoli and Cucumber Juice

Ingredients for the Kiwi, Pineapple, Broccoli and Cucumber Juice

- 1 peeled and chopped kiwi

- 1-2 cups of pineapple chunks

- 1 cucumber slices

- 1/3 cups of chopped broccoli

Preparing the juice:

1. Carefully remove the peel of the ingredients and chop them into smaller pieces.

2. Blend the ingredients together in a juicer and pour the drink in a glass.

3. Add ice cubes and enjoy.

How does it help me reduce weight?

Pineapples offer enzyme rich nutrition that detoxifies your body and allows you flush out the toxins. The four ingredients act together to provide a high energy drinks that is essential for your physical endurance.

Lemon, Apple, Red Leaf Lettuce and Cucumber Juice

Ingredients for the Lemon, Apple, Red Leaf Lettuce and Cucumber Juice

- 1 apple

- 1lemon fruit

- 5 leaves of red leaf lettuce

- 1-2 cucumbers

Preparing the juice:

1. Rinse the ingredients thoroughly.

2. Slice the apple and cucumbers into wedges (do not remove the outer layer or the skin.)

3. Peel the lemon and remove all the seeds. Seeds never blend properly and do not offer any substantial benefit.

4. Tear the lettuce leaves into small pieces.

5. Blend all the ingredients in the juicer and have a nourishing drink.

How does it help me reduce weight?

Red leaf lettuce is one of the most nourishing leafy vegetables. It is rich in calcium, vitamins (A and K), iron and other important nutrients that help you build body strength. Lettuce helps your metabolism and immune system. This recipe can be a great after - work out drink.

Cucumber, Apple, Carrots and Celery Juice

Ingredients for the Cucumber, Apple, Carrots and Celery Juice

- 4-5 red apples

- 1-2 small cucumbers

- 1 large carrot

- 2-3 celery stalks

Preparing the juice:

1. Rinse all the ingredients thoroughly with water before use. Pay extra attention to the carrots as they can have dirt and soil in their skin.

2. Slice the apples in four pieces.

3. Avoid peeling the cucumber. Just like apple peel, cucumber peel also contains nutrients that can contribute positively towards your physical health.

4. Blend all the ingredients in the juicer and enjoy a healthy, refreshing drink.

How does it help me reduce weight?

As mentioned above, cucumber, apples and celery contain high level of nutrients that not provide physical strength, but also reduce fat deposits in the body. The combination of these four ingredients ensures that get the right amount of calories during the day for better performance.

Apple, Kale, Lettuce, Celery and Cucumber Juice

Ingredients for the Apple, Kale, Lettuce, Celery and Cucumber Juice

- 1 -2 apples

- 3-4 large kale leaves

- 2-3 large lettuce leaves

- 2-3 celery stalks

- 1 cucumber

Preparing the juice:

1. After washing the ingredients.

2. Peel off the cucumber skin and chop into slices

3. Cut the celery stalks into smaller pieces

4. Combine all the ingredients in the juicer and blend.

5. You will notice a unique green color that would be the result of kale and lettuce.

6. Pour the drink in your favorite and consume before or after exercise for higher physical endurance.

How does it help me reduce weight?

Vegetables like kale, celery and lettuce provide countless vitamins and antioxidants that are necessary for your overall health. When you work out, your body works double than it usually does, which is why you need a proper nutrition for high endurance.

It is important to remember that the above-mentioned juice recipes are meant to cure any obesity problems; the drinks will not help you lose substantial weight within weeks. However, the drinks will help you gain the strength that you need to get through your weight loss goals.

The purpose of the above recipes is to provide you the fruit and vegetable combinations that can act fast to provide the antioxidants and other nutrition that is important for the physical fortitude. It is very crucial that you understand the nutritional value of all the ingredients before you consume them. If you are diabetic, then do not, under any circumstance, use more fruit for the juices. For diabetic people, vegetable combinations will work best.

Moreover, make sure that you are not allergic to any of the ingredients mentioned above. Some of the fruits can cause serious allergies in some people, so make sure that you are fully aware of the ingredients and their properties.

Ancient Recipes for Weight Loss

There are many proven recipes that make you lose weight very fast and they also help you keep that weight off. This is how the people in the past stayed healthy and kept their own bodies toned before things such as supplements, gyms and other such methods were either discovered or invented. Here are a number of ancient recipes that will help you lose weight.

Hot Water and Lemon for Weight Loss

Hot water and lemon are two of the most effective ingredients in losing weight. Lemon works very effectively by cutting the grease and the fats that have been stored in the body. Hot water also serves the same function. When you combine lemon in hot water you can flush out all the toxic materials in your body and say hello to good and healthy weight loss. Not only that, lemon juice is inclusive of Calcium, pectin fiber, Vitamin C and Potassium. When you receive all these nutritional benefits in something that is less than 25 calories you benefit greatly from consuming it. It can also balance the pH levels in the human body.

If you want to prepare lemon and hot water all you have to do is boil a cup of water, let it cool a little until you think you can drink it and then squeeze the juice of one lemon in it. You will find that it will benefit you greatly. The best thing about this is that it is very easy to drink.

Hot and Cold Water for Weight Loss

Many people in Japan adopt the practice of taking a bath in hot and cold water simultaneously in order to lose weight and to become relaxed or to make themselves alert. They have an abundance of hot springs in Japan, in which they have conducted such experiments which are good for the muscles in your body. Following this practice is fairly simple and it allows you to relax your muscles and make your brain alert in an effective manner. All you have to do is:

- Take a relaxing bath with warm water in the tub so that your muscles become relaxed and the body's immune system becomes stronger.

- Immediately after this take a cold shower or a cold bath so that the body can transition

- Take another warm bath

- Take another cold bath or shower

If you wish to keep or make your mind alert then it is best to take a cold shower or a bath at the end however, if you wish to be relaxed after the bath then it is best to finish with a warm bath instead.

Oolong Tea for Weight Loss

Oolong tea is a great type of weight loss tea that is also commonly referred to as Chinese oolong tea, wu-long tea or brown tea. In Asian countries the role of tea in losing weight and keeping it off is very much essential. It is very well known as a concoction that decreases the stored fat inside the body. It also works by speeding up the metabolism. Another benefit of the oolong tea is that it blocks fat from storing themselves in the body by building new enzymes that keep the fat away.

Some people are of the belief that it is even more effective than green tea. Here are some benefits of Oolong tea that you probably did not know about.

- It contains many anti-oxidants that can kick start your metabolism b 10%. These are helpful in burning fats and help you lose weight.

- It can protect you from many chronic diseases. By drinking oolong tea you develop a very healthy immune system.

- Oolong tea blocks fat by building enzymes and prevents them from entering the body and being stored in it.

- It regulates the blood sugar levels and makes you feel satisfied. You do not crave sweets when you consume oolong tea.

- It contains negative calories which help you become thin.

You must have at least two cups of oolong tea every single day so that you can lose weight. You can prepare oolong tea in the following way:

- Boil a cup of hot water and add one teaspoon of oolong tea powder in it.

- Stir the oolong tea in the boiling water for as long as ten to fifteen minutes.

- Strain it and then cool a little bit of the tea before taking a sip

- Enjoy the tea

Weight Loss with Kefir

Kefir is a very well-known substance that is famously known for reducing lactose intolerance by 50%. It reduces the flatulence effect and also cuts the calories in the lactose and prevents them from being stored in the body. The most important feature of Kefir is the fact that it contains a fatty acid by the name of Conjugated linoleic acid which is popularly known to reduce the fat in the body and increase metabolic activity. This means that the digestive system becomes active and ends up burning the fat that the body consumes.

You need to have a proper and working digestive system in order to lose weight and most importantly, to keep the weight off. It is very much easier to lose weight than to keep it off for a long period of time. Kefir is a dairy product that helps you do that and it is even more beneficial than yogurt in this regard.

Kefir has a special enzyme in it which enables it to digest lactose. This means that even if you are a person who likes to consume dairy products but gain a lot of weight from it you need to start consuming Kefir so that it can cut the calories in lactose and make you slim, just the way you want it to.

Conclusion

For many people it is of extreme importance to lose weight but they find it nearly impossible to do something without abandoning the idea or cursing themselves. They find it hard to continue with one type of diet and when they fail, they completely give up on the idea of a thin body.

However, losing weight is not just the idea of becoming thin and having a toned body. It goes a lot farther than that. It means incorporating a few changes into your lifestyle which enable you to stay healthy and toned and slim and fit. This means that you need to be healthy before you can become thin. When it really comes down to it, anybody can completely starve themselves, go on a crash diet and lose a bunch of weight. They still cannot continue that for long (and neither should they) and there comes a time when they come back to their regular eating habits.

They either come back to their old eating habits or they can become anorexic which makes it even worse. Instead of having an eating disorder or some other health complication, maybe you should adopt a healthier, safer and more effective way of losing weight. You should opt for a diet that is actually good for your body, gives you plenty of good nutrients and keeps you away from the bad fats and the calories.

In addition to that, there is also the big factor of exercise. Many people believe that they can cut down on the amount of food that they eat if they avoid exercise. However, that is completely untrue because when you exercise your body is molded into the shape you want to see it in. You can actually see the supple layers of your muscles coming into shape and your limbs and your tummy forming into the shape you want to see them in. You cannot have an even and toned supple body without putting it through the process of exercise. You may starve yourself, go on a diet or anything of the sort but you will not be able to tone the muscles. They will only get rid of the fats stored inside them and that will be the end of that.

When you diet and exercise, you also have to remember that a great role is played by your mind in the whole process. You cannot ignore the benefits of positive thinking when it comes to transitioning something this important in your life. You have to understand that your brain plays as important a role as any in this whole procedure. When you think positive thoughts and make yourself determined to accomplish this goal, there is no one who can stop you from achieving the goal of perfect weight.

You can also derive some wisdom and benefits from ancient weight loss recipes such as hot water and lemon and even oolong tea. These types of things can be your aid in the quest to lose weight and to become healthy and fit. You cannot be thin for long until you are really driven to do it, so keep your mind on it and set on the journey to lose weight today!

Special gift for readers

Throughout the book, there are numerous mentions of additional resources that can help you through this journey. You can get all these valuable resources by visiting our website www.puredietweightloss.com/newsletter

You can also join our mailing list and get updates on new releases, free mini-courses, and new recipes we introduce from time to time based on our research. Click here to sign up.